Health Care Provider CPR

Art Breault RN, AEMT-P/FF, NREMT-P
Medical Writer

Stephen J. Rahm, NREMT-P
EMS Professions Educator

Benjamin Gulli, MD
Medical Editor

Jon R. Krohmer, MD, FACEP
Medical Editor

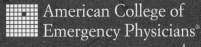

American College of
Emergency Physicians®

ADVANCING EMERGENCY CARE

JONES AND BARTLETT PUBLISHERS

Sudbury, Massachusetts

BOSTON   TORONTO   LONDON   SINGAPORE

Jones and Bartlett Publishers

World Headquarters
40 Tall Pine Drive
Sudbury, MA 01776
info@jbpub.com
www.ECSInstitute.org

Jones and Bartlett Publishers Canada
6339 Ormindale Way
Mississauga, Ontario L5V 1J2
Canada

Jones and Bartlett Publishers International
Barb House, Barb Mews
London W6 7PA
United Kingdom

Jones and Bartlett's books and products are available through most bookstores and online booksellers. To contact Jones and Bartlett Publishers directly, call 800-832-0034, fax 978-443-8000, or visit our website www.jbpub.com.

Substantial discounts on bulk quantities of Jones and Bartlett's publications are available to corporations, professional associations, and other qualified organizations. For details and specific discount information, contact the special sales department at Jones and Bartlett via the above contact information or send an email to specialsales@jbpub.com.

Production Credits
Chief Executive Officer: Clayton Jones
Chief Operating Officer: Donald W. Jones, Jr
President, Higher Education and Professional Publishing: Robert Holland
V.P., Sales and Marketing: William J. Kane
V.P., Production and Design: Anne Spencer
V.P., Manufacturing and Inventory Control: Therese Connell
Publisher, Public Safety: Kimberly Brophy
Acquisitions Editor: Christine Emerton

AAOS

AMERICAN ACADEMY OF
ORTHOPAEDIC SURGEONS

Editorial Credits
Chief Education Officer: Mark W. Wieting
Director, Department of Publications: Marilyn L. Fox, PhD
Managing Editor: Barbara A. Scotese
Associate Senior Editor: Gayle Murray

AAOS Board of Directors 2007
James H. Beaty, MD
E. Anthony Rankin, MD
Joseph D. Zuckerman, MD
William L. Healy, MD
Thomas C. Barber, MD
Kevin J. Bozic, MD, MBA
John T. Gill, MD
Christopher D. Harner, MD
Richard F. Kyle, MD
Joseph C. McCarthy, MD
Norman Y. Otsuka, MD
William J. Robb III, MD
Matthew S. Shapiro, MD
James P. Tasto, MD
G. Zachary Wilhoit, MS, MBA
Ken Yamaguchi, MD
Karen L. Hackett, *FACHE, CAE (Ex officio)*

Senior Production Editor: Susan Schultz
Photo Research Manager/Photographer: Kimberly Potvin
Director of Marketing: Alisha Weisman
Interior Design: Anne Spencer
Cover Design: Kristin E. Ohlin
Composition: Shepherd Inc.
Text Printing and Binding: Courier
Cover Printing: Courier
Cover Photograph: © Jones and Bartlett Publishers. Courtesy of MIEMSS.

Library of Congress Cataloging-in-Publication Data
Health care provider CPR / Art Breault ... [et al.].
   p. ; cm.
  Includes index.
  ISBN 978-0-7637-5593-5 (pbk)
  1. CPR (First aid)—Handbooks, manuals, etc. I. Breault, Art.
  [DNLM: 1. Cardiopulmonary Resuscitation—methods—Handbooks. WG 39 H434 2008]
  RC87.9.H39 2008
  616.1′025—dc22

                2007040124

6048

Additional photographic and illustration credits appear on page 90, which constitutes a continuation of the copyright page.
11 10 09 08 07   10 9 8 7 6 5 4 3 2 1

contents

welcome

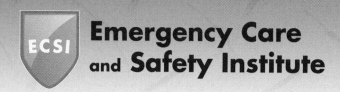

Emergency Care and **Safety Institute**

Welcome to the Emergency Care and Safety Institute

Welcome to the Emergency Care and Safety Institute (ECSI), brought to you by the American Academy of Orthopaedic Surgeons (AAOS) and the American College of Emergency Physicians (ACEP).

The ECSI is an educational organization created for the purpose of delivering the highest quality training to laypersons and professionals in the areas of First Aid, CPR, AED, Bloodborne Pathogens, and related safety and health fields.

Two of the most respected names in injury, illness, and emergency medical care—the AAOS and the ACEP—have approved the content in our training materials.

AAOS
AMERICAN ACADEMY OF
ORTHOPAEDIC SURGEONS

About the AAOS

The AAOS provides education and practice management services for orthopaedic surgeons and allied health professionals. The AAOS also serves as an advocate for improved patient care and informs the public about the science of orthopaedics. Founded in 1933, the not-for-profit AAOS has grown from a small organization serving less than 500 members to the world's largest medical association of musculoskeletal specialists. The AAOS now serves about 24,000 members internationally.

American College of
Emergency Physicians®

ADVANCING EMERGENCY CARE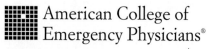

About ACEP

ACEP was founded in 1968 and is the world's oldest and largest emergency medicine specialty organization. Today it represents more than 22,000 members and is the emergency medicine specialty society recognized as the acknowledged leader in emergency medicine.

ECSI Course Catalog

Individuals seeking training in ECSI subjects can choose from among various online and offline course offerings. The following courses are available through the ECSI:

First Aid, CPR, and AED Standard

CPR and AED

Professional Rescuer CPR

Health Care Provider CPR

First Aid

Wilderness First Aid

Bloodborne Pathogens

First Responder

First Aid and CPR Online

First Aid Online

Adult CPR Online

Adult and Pediatric CPR Online

Professional Rescuer CPR Online

AED Online

Adult CPR and AED Online

Bloodborne Pathogens Online

The ECSI offers a wide range of textbooks, instructor and student support materials, and interactive technology, including online courses. Every ECSI textbook is the center of an integrated teaching and learning system that offers instructor, student, and technology resources to better support instructors and prepare students. The instructor supplements provide practical hands-on, time-saving tools like PowerPoint presentations, DVDs, and web-based distance learning resources. The student supplements are designed to help students retain the most important information and to assist them in preparing for exams. And, a key component to the teaching and learning systems are technology resources that provide interactive exercises and simulations to help students become great emergency responders.

Documents attesting to the ECSI's recognitions of satisfactory course completion will be issued to those who successfully meet the course objectives and criteria for passing the course. Written acknowledgement of a participant's successful course completion is provided in the form of a Course Completion Card, issued by the ECSI.

Visit www.ECSInstitute.org today!

resource preview

This textbook is designed to give health care professionals the education and confidence they need to effectively provide emergency care. Features that reinforce and expand on essential information include:

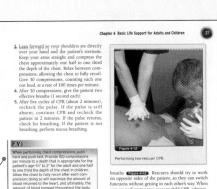

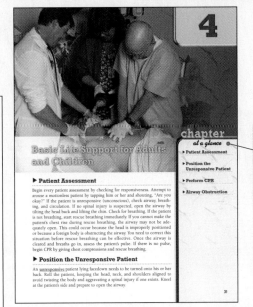

Chapter at a Glance
Guides students through the key topics covered in that chapter.

FYI Boxes
Include valuable information related to the injuries or illnesses discussed in that section, including prevention tips and risk factors.

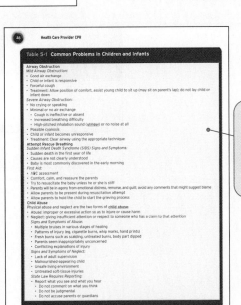

Tables
Provide a concise summary of critical medical information related to the chapter topic.

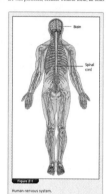

Chapter 2 Understanding the Human Body 15

stimulation, and the nervous system controls movement. Signals travel from the brain through a network of nerves that extend down the spinal cord and branch out through the body. These nerves act much like transistor circuits, sending and receiving messages at an incredible rate of speed. Figure 2-1.

Structure and Function

The brain and spinal cord serve as the headquarters and communication system for the body. They are well protected, because without them, all other systems would fail. The brain is encased in the skull, and the spinal cord is inside the vertebrae of the spine.

The spinal cord can be thought of as the main circuit board of a communication system. It relays sensory information from peripheral nerves to the brain and forwards signals from the brain to the body through motor fibers. Injury to any area of the spinal cord can disrupt the flow of information to and from the brain.

The brain has three main parts: the cerebrum (large portion of the brain), the cerebellum (small portion of the brain), and the brain stem. Figure 2-2. The cerebrum controls thought, sensation, memory, and voluntary motions such as walking or picking up an object. The cerebellum is located at the back of the head and below the cerebrum. It controls balance by coordinating signals from the eyes and inner ears. The medulla oblongata, located in the brain stem, connects the cerebrum and the cerebellum to the spinal cord. It controls involuntary motions, such as breathing, heart rate, and digestion.

Of all the organs and tissues in the body, the brain is particularly sensitive to oxygen deprivation. When either the respiratory or circulatory system fails, cells in the brain begin to die in as little as 4 to 6 minutes because of the lack of oxygen. Rescue breathing and CPR can help keep the brain oxygenated until the patient can receive specialized medical care.

Figure 2-1   Human nervous system.

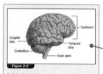

Figure 2-2   Surface of the brain.

Vocabulary
Key terms highlighted and defined throughout the text.

Color Photographs and Artwork
Illustrate processes, devices, and rescue methods described in the text.

---

prep kit 77

▶ **Ready for Review**

- Special resuscitation situations include trauma, drowning, hypothermia, and electric shock. These situations present you with special challenges when providing care. Remember that trauma victims may have sustained spinal injuries, which require you to immobilize the entire spinal column.

- When water rescue is needed, you should attempt it in this order: reach, throw, row, and go. Never attempt a water rescue unless you have special training and equipment for this type of rescue. Consider the possibility of spinal injury in anyone found unresponsive in the water, especially shallow water. Clear the patient's airway before beginning resuscitation. Unless obvious signs of death are present, attempt resuscitation—even if the victim has been submerged for a prolonged period of time. This is especially true if the patient was rescued from cold water.

- Hypothermia may occur with patients who have been submerged in cool or cold water, and in other situations besides extreme cold weather. Because severe hypothermia dramatically slows the heart rate and breathing, assess the patient's breathing and pulse for 30 to 45 seconds before initiating CPR. Handle the hypothermic patient gently; they are at greater risk for cardiac arrest.

- When dealing with electric shock, make sure there is no longer any danger of electrocution. Your first consideration is your own safety. Do not attempt to gain access to the patient until the scene is safe. Assume that patients may have serious internal injuries, even if entrance and exit wounds are small. Because electrocution injuries cause massive muscle spasms, you should also suspect a spinal injury.

▶ **Vital Vocabulary**

drowning Submersion in water resulting in death within 24 hours.

hypothermia An abnormally low body temperature.

near drowning Survival, at least for more than 24 hours, following submersion in water.

▶ **Check Your Knowledge**

1. To have the best chance for survival, a patient with serious trauma must:
   A. have blankets applied to him or her.
   B. be transported to a trauma center.
   C. receive oxygen as soon as possible.
   D. receive early care by paramedics.

2. Before attempting any water rescue, you should:
   A. take precautions to ensure your own safety.
   B. ask the patient if he or she can swim to shore.
   C. determine how long the patient has been in the water.
   D. have paramedics standing by so ALS care can be provided.

3. Severe hypothermia is characterized by all of the following, EXCEPT:
   A. a core body temperature of less than 86°F (30°C).
   B. severe disorientation or unresponsiveness.
   C. a lack of shivering as body temperature drops.
   D. relaxed, flaccid muscles due to a lack of oxygen.

4. The first thing you should do when caring for a hypothermic patient is:
   A. check for a pulse for 30 to 45 seconds.
   B. open the patient's airway with the jaw-thrust maneuver.
   C. carefully move the patient to a warmer area.
   D. complete a full head-to-toe assessment.

Prep Kit
End-of-chapter activities reinforce important concepts and improve students' comprehension.
- **Ready for Review:** Thoroughly summarizes chapter content.
- **Vital Vocabulary:** Lists the key terms and definitions from the chapter.
- **Check Your Knowledge:** Quizzes students on the chapter's core concepts.

78

appendix   **Evaluation Forms**

Student's Name: _____   Date: _____

One-Rescuer Adult and Child CPR Steps

No.	Task Steps	Satisfactory	Unsatisfactory
1.	Check responsiveness.		
2.	If unresponsive, activate the EMS system.		
3.	Open the airway (head tilt–chin lift or jaw-thrust).		
4.	Check for breathing. Look, listen, and feel for at least 5 seconds but no longer than 10 seconds.		
5.	If not breathing, give two breaths (1 second per breath).		
6.	If breaths produce visible chest rise, check circulation (carotid pulse, movement, coughing).		
7.	If circulation is present, but breathing is absent, perform rescue breathing (one breath every 5 to 6 seconds for an adult; one breath every 3 to 5 seconds for a child).		
8.	If no circulation, give 30 chest compressions (rate of 100 chest compressions per minute) and two breaths (1 second per breath).		
9.	After five cycles (about 2 minutes) of CPR, recheck circulation. If no circulation, continue CPR and recheck circulation every 2 minutes.		
10.	If alone and the patient is a child, call 9-1-1 (if not already done) after five cycles (about 2 minutes) of CPR. Then return to the child and continue CPR.		

Retest Approved By: _____   Retest Evaluator: _____

Evaluation Forms
Evaluation forms for step-by-step testing.

Acknowledgments

Jones and Bartlett Publishers would like to thank the following people for their expert review of the text:

Carol Boswell, EdD, RN, CNE, FANE
Professor and Co-director
Center of Excellence in Evidence-Based Practice
Texas Tech University Health Sciences Center
Odessa, Texas

Roberta Kaplow, RN, PhD, CCNS, CCRN
Clinical Nurse Educator
Atlanta, Georgia

Donamarie N. Wilfong, MSN, RN, DNP Candidate
Director of Clinical Operations
The STAR Center for Simulation, Teaching, Academics, and Research
Western Pennsylvania Hospital
Pittsburgh, Pennsylvania

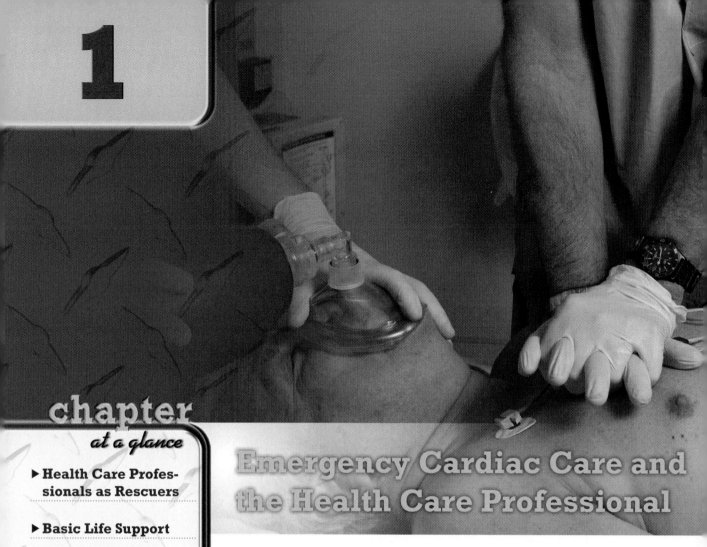

Emergency Cardiac Care and the Health Care Professional

▶ Health Care Professionals as Rescuers

Health care professionals, physicians, and physician assistants will likely participate in many cardiac arrest "codes" during their careers, not only while on duty but also potentially in other places in the community. The cause of the cardiac arrest may be ventricular fibrillation, acute myocardial infarction, poisoning, cerebral vascular accident, or trauma, among others.

Most cardiac arrests are not witnessed by health care professionals working in the community, ambulatory setting, or other unmonitored unit; they almost always occur before a health care professional arrives on the scene or reaches the patient's bedside. When at work, health care professionals should follow both the national guidelines and their local protocols for providing basic and advanced cardiac life support.

▶ Basic Life Support

The initial care that the health care professional provides is known as basic life support (BLS), which plays an important role in the outcome of a patient. Three of the most important basic life support skills are:

  ○ Rescue breathing—provided when someone has stopped breathing
    Figure 1-1

- Cardiopulmonary resuscitation (CPR)—provided when someone's heart has stopped beating **Figure 1-2**
- Abdominal thrusts (Heimlich maneuver)—provided when someone is conscious and has an airway obstruction (choking) **Figure 1-3**

This text covers these and other skills used to care for victims of respiratory and cardiac emergencies. It also covers special situations you are likely to encounter and the use of specialized equipment, most notably automated external defibrillators (AEDs) **Figure 1-4** .

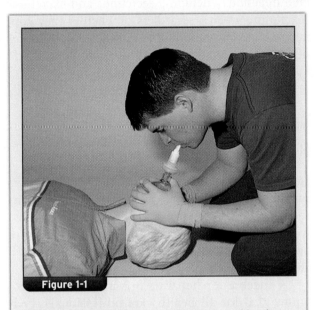

Figure 1-1

Seal your mouth over the mouthpiece and begin rescue breathing.

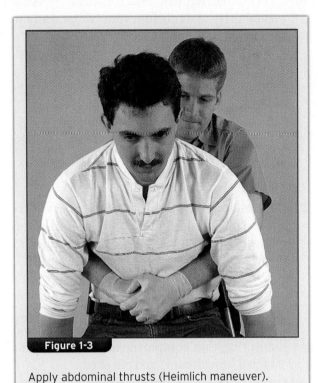

Figure 1-3

Apply abdominal thrusts (Heimlich maneuver).

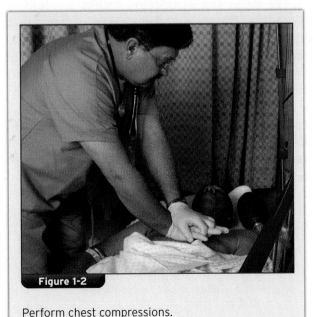

Figure 1-2

Perform chest compressions.

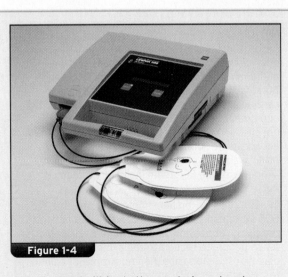

Figure 1-4

AEDs have a built-in rhythm analysis system to determine whether the victim needs to be shocked.

▶ Preparing for Emergencies

As a health care provider, you need to prepare for an emergency in advance. Reading this text and taking a CPR course are only the first steps in preparing for the various emergency situations you could encounter. You will need additional physical and mental preparation before you will be ready to provide emergency care. This includes:

- Being physically fit for the strenuous work you will perform.
- Being mentally prepared for the challenges you could face.
- Periodically reviewing your skills and rehearsing your response with other professional rescuers and health care providers.
- Practicing with the equipment and supplies you will be using.
- Examining additional reference material, as it becomes available, to stay up-to-date on changes in CPR techniques and advances in care.
- Being prepared for the personal risks associated with your job, such as the possibility of injury or disease transmission.
- Being prepared by restocking supplies and ensuring that equipment is properly maintained, functioning, and checked.

FYI

Emergency Cardiac Care

In some instances, the level of emergency cardiac care (ECC) that you provide may require additional education or certification. This education may include advances in the treatment of cardiac and respiratory arrest, the use of specific equipment designed for either hospital or non-hospital settings, and an understanding of advanced life support (ALS) techniques used by other members of the emergency care team. Members of the ECC team include paramedics, nurses, physician assistants, and physicians.

In addition, you can help implement an effective ECC system in your community. You can educate the public about how to prevent heart disease, teach people to recognize the symptoms of cardiac arrest, emphasize the importance of calling for assistance (9-1-1), and encourage others to learn basic life support skills, such as CPR.

▶ Disease Transmission and Precautions

As a health care professional, you must be aware of the risks of disease transmission associated with emergency care. All bodily fluids should be considered infectious, including secretions and excretions (excluding sweat), regardless of whether they contain blood. The bloodborne and airborne diseases of particular concern to health care providers are:

- Hepatitis B and C (bloodborne).
- Human immunodeficiency virus (HIV) (bloodborne).
- Tuberculosis (airborne).

Hepatitis

Hepatitis is a viral infection of the liver. The virus can stay in the liver and cause severe damage (cirrhosis) and cancer. Hepatitis B and C are most worrisome to health care providers. Each type of hepatitis is caused by a different virus. Hepatitis B affects more than 100,000 people each year.

A vaccine for hepatitis B is available and recommended for all health care professionals. Federal laws require employers to offer the vaccine to employees who may be at risk of exposure. Individuals who have not received the vaccine and who are exposed to hepatitis B may begin to experience signs and symptoms within 2 weeks to 6 months. The signs and symptoms of hepatitis B resemble those of the flu and include fatigue, nausea, loss of appetite, stomach pain, and jaundice (yellowing of the skin). Although some people with hepatitis B may not have the usual signs and symptoms, they can still infect others who are exposed to their blood. Like hepatitis B, hepatitis C can also lead to long-term liver disease, including cancer. However, there is currently no vaccine or effective treatment for hepatitis C.

FYI

Hepatitis B Vaccine

The hepatitis B vaccine is more than 96% effective in individuals completing the three-shot immunization series.

Human Immunodeficiency Virus

Human immunodeficiency virus, commonly called HIV, attacks white blood cells and destroys the body's ability to fight infection. AIDS (acquired immunodeficiency syndrome) is a result of HIV infection. Like hepatitis, HIV is transmitted through contact with blood or blood components. There are more than 400,000 people in the United States infected with HIV; at present, AIDS is always fatal. Because there is no HIV vaccine, the best defense is to avoid direct contact with blood.

Tuberculosis

Airborne diseases are viruses and bacteria introduced into the air by coughing or sneezing. Tuberculosis (TB) is a serious disease that affects the respiratory system. It is caused by bacteria that settle in the lungs. The signs and symptoms of TB include coughing, fatigue, weight loss, chest pain, and coughing up blood. A strain of TB known as multidrug-resistant TB has been identified. This strain developed when TB patients failed to complete prescribed antibiotic treatment. Remaining bacteria became resistant to the antibiotic, and the patient suffers a relapse as the bacteria spread.

Protection

Standard precautions means creating a barrier between you and the victim with personal protective equipment (PPE). You must anticipate contact with bodily fluids. The PPE you have available to you when dealing with a cardiac or respiratory emergency includes:

- Eye protection, such as goggles or eyeglasses with side shields.
- Medical exam gloves such as vinyl or nitrile gloves.
- Mouth-to-barrier devices for rescue breathing **Figure 1-5**.
- Antiseptic wipes or solution for washing your hands immediately after providing care.

When responding to an emergency in the community, you may need to improvise with equipment that is readily available, such as plastic bags, soap, and hand sanitizers.

As a health care professional, you are eligible to receive vaccinations against certain types of dis-

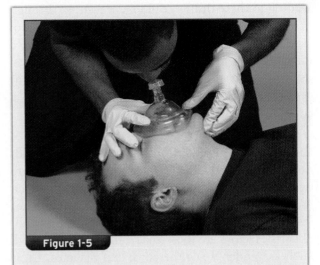

Figure 1-5

A barrier device is an essential component of your personal protective equipment.

ease as outlined by federal and state Occupational Safety and Health Administration (OSHA) regulations. Your employer is also required to establish work practices and engineering controls to help prevent the likelihood of disease transmission. A copy of these plans and practices should be made available to you. OSHA's regulations apply to those individuals who are designated or expected to render care as part of their job. They exclude unassigned employees who provide unanticipated care.

▶ Cardiovascular Disease: Improving the Odds

Cardiovascular disease (CVD) is the leading cause of death in the United States. According to the American Heart Association, CVD accounts for more than 900,000 deaths each year. Of these, more than 400,000 are attributed to coronary heart disease (CHD). Each year more than 225,000 people die of CHD within 1 hour of the onset of the signs and symptoms and before reaching the hospital.* These are known as sudden deaths from cardiac arrest. Although the death rate from CVD has been declining slightly, there is still much room for improvement. Many of the causes

*Source: American Heart Association. 2006 Heart and Stroke Statistical Update.

leading to these deaths could be prevented through a heart-healthy lifestyle that reduces the risks of heart disease. As a health care provider, you have an obligation to reduce your personal risk factors, as well as to educate others so that they might reduce their risk factors.

Risk Factors

Risk factors for CVD fall into two categories: avoidable and unavoidable. Avoidable risk factors are behaviors or conditions that can be controlled, such as cigarette smoking, high blood pressure, high cholesterol, lack of exercise, stress, and obesity. Unavoidable risk factors are those that cannot be controlled, such as gender, aging, heredity, and diabetes. Cigarette smokers are much more likely to develop CVD, suffer a heart attack, or have a stroke than nonsmokers are. The risk increases with the number of cigarettes smoked, and decreases and even may be eliminated if the smoker stops smoking.

High blood pressure, left untreated or uncontrolled, significantly increases the chances of coronary artery disease and is a major risk factor for stroke. Fortunately, there are a variety of medications available to control high blood pressure.

High cholesterol can result from a diet high in saturated fats and from hereditary factors. A fatty diet has been associated with the development of fatty deposits on the artery walls (atherosclerosis). Countries such as the United States, where the average person's diet is high in saturated fats, have correspondingly high rates of coronary artery disease.

Lack of exercise and a sedentary lifestyle make the body ill-prepared for physically demanding tasks that can raise a person's heart rate above tolerable levels and increase stress on the heart. Obesity is also a high-risk factor, not only because it is often associated with poor diet and lack of exercise, but also because excessive weight strains the heart.

Prevention: Heart-Healthy Living

A commitment to a heart-healthy lifestyle is the best way to prevent cardiovascular disease and heart attack. The basics of heart-healthy living are easy to remember and simple to teach to others. As a professional rescuer, you are responsible for educating others about prevention practices and for being a role model to others by practicing these yourself.

- Stop smoking, if you have not already done so, and urge others to stop.
- Exercise regularly. A brisk, 15- to 30-minute walk every day provides excellent aerobic conditioning.
- Eat a healthy, balanced diet, low in sodium and saturated fat.
- Have your blood pressure checked regularly, and take prescribed medication for high blood pressure.

▶ The Chain of Survival

It is possible to reduce the number of deaths from heart disease through a Chain of Survival Figure 1-6 . This chain has four links: early access, early CPR, early defibrillation, and early Advanced Cardiac Life Support (ACLS).

Early Access to Care

Early access to the emergency medical service (EMS) is the first critical link in the Chain of Survival. In the event of a respiratory or cardiac emergency, access the EMS system by calling 9-1-1 (in most areas). The 9-1-1 system covers approximately 85% of the U.S. population. Those without 9-1-1 service must access EMS by calling their local 7-digit emergency number. A prompt call will ensure the timely arrival of EMS personnel with the necessary training and equipment to provide appropriate care. You should know your local EMS system activation number in your area. Plan ahead.

Dispatchers who take calls should be trained to recognize symptoms of respiratory and cardiac emergencies. This will allow them to provide prearrival instructions to callers over the phone and start early advanced or tiered ALS response. In addition to instructing a caller on how to perform CPR and to remove an airway obstruction, dispatchers should advise patients with no history of aspirin allergy or signs of active or recent gastrointestinal bleeding to chew 160 to 325 mg of aspirin. Early administration of aspirin has clearly proven to be effective in reducing mortality from a cardiac event.

EMS systems are composed of professionals who provide skilled emergency care to people who are ill or injured. This includes providing emergency cardiac care, such as CPR. These professionals share

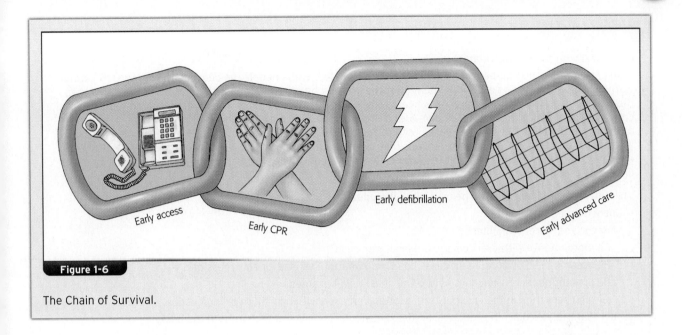

Figure 1-6

The Chain of Survival.

Early access

Early CPR

Early defibrillation

Early advanced care

a defined duty to respond to an emergency. They are found in a broad range of health care, allied health care, and nonmedical settings **Figure 1-7** .

Examples of personnel who function as professional rescuers include:

- Fire fighters.
- Law enforcement officers.
- First responders, emergency medical technicians, and paramedics.
- Nurses, physician assistants, and physicians.
- Occupational or physical therapists, lab technicians, and radiologists.
- Athletic trainers.
- Military personnel.
- Industrial and business personnel.
- Park services personnel.
- Ski patrol members.
- Lifeguards.
- Airline personnel.
- Cruise ship personnel.

Early CPR

When a person's heart stops beating, <u>cardiopulmonary resuscitation (CPR)</u> is needed. CPR temporarily helps circulate oxygenated blood throughout the body. This lessens the chance of brain damage and increases the chance of survival, especially when CPR is coupled with early defibrillation. To be most effective, CPR must be started

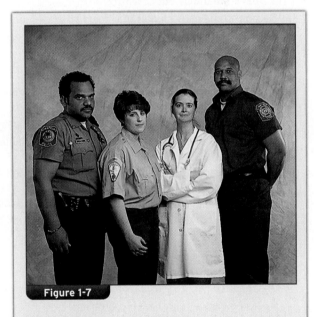

Figure 1-7

Professional rescuers include experts from many fields; among them are EMTs, fire fighters, law enforcement officials, and physicians.

promptly and properly. Each minute of delay reduces the chance of survival. *Interruptions of CPR should be limited as much as possible.* Advanced procedures, advanced airways, medications, and rhythm checks should be planned to allow for maximum compression time.

FYI

Early Warning Signs of a Heart Attack

Heart attacks are the number-one killer in the United States. Some people die because they ignore the early warning signals of a heart attack and deny that these could be life-threatening signs. Most of the damage to the heart occurs in the first 2 hours of a heart attack. For this reason, heart attack victims need rapid medical care to help minimize the amount of damage to the heart. But because the early warning signals of a heart attack are often mild, they are not easily recognized by laypersons as potentially fatal, and people delay seeking the necessary care. Part of your responsibility as a health care provider and a professional rescuer is to educate community members about the importance of recognizing a heart attack in its early stages so that immediate action can be taken to save more lives.

The early warning signals of a heart attack include:
- Chest discomfort that may:
  - Recur and increase in intensity.
  - Be more intense with exertion and diminish with rest.
  - Be accompanied by light-headedness, fainting, sweating, nausea, or shortness of breath.
  - Be present hours or even days before the chest pain becomes severe.
- A burning sensation in the chest or throat (often confused with heartburn or indigestion).
- Pain that radiates down the left arm, across the shoulders, jaw, and neck, or into the back.

The public should be educated to:
- Recognize the early signals of a heart attack in another person and intervene.
- Convince a family member, friend, coworker, or even a stranger who exhibits signs of a heart attack that medical care is needed immediately.
- Move from being passive observers and listeners to active early heart attack care providers.

As professionals, you can use these key points to educate people in your community and encourage them to action:
- The progression of a heart attack can be halted if people are alert to the early signals and actively intervene.
- It makes sense to have mild chest discomfort evaluated before a complete blockage takes place and damages the heart.
- Once the heart stops, it may be shocked into action through defibrillation. But by this time, heart damage has already occurred and sometimes death cannot be averted.
- Denial and delay are common among victims and are often reinforced by those around the victim. This occurs because the reality of a heart attack is too traumatic to face.
  - A heart attack poses serious short- and long-term inconveniences to the victim and the victim's family.
  - A heart attack is inconsistent with the victim's self-perception or the bystander's perceptions of the victim.
  - A heart attack is something that happens to others, not to the victim.
- Use the acronym ACT WISELY to teach others how to intervene:
  A Acknowledge that there is a problem.
  C Calmly assess the situation and persuade the victim to get help.
  T Tenacity. Be persistent, and do not give in.
  W Willingness to act.
  I Influence, and use your skills creatively.
  S Simplify the discussion and decisions.
  E Empathy. Understand why the victim is resisting help.
  L Link the victim with the nearest hospital.
  Y "Yes, I will get help!" Get the victim to state this.

FYI

- Learn how to set up an early defibrillation program
  - Properly deployed, AEDs save additional patients' lives, inside the hospital as well as in the community.
  - AHA Class I recommendation for a collapse-to-shock interval of less than 3 minutes in all areas of hospital and ambulatory care facilities. Time recognizing cardiac arrest and delivering first shock can vary significantly across patient care units.
  - Focus on ease of use, portability, and maintenance when selecting AED devices.
  - Placement of AEDs within a 3-minute brisk walk: Outlying areas such as outpatient clinics and rehabilitation centers.
  - Knowledge of current state AED legislation.
  - Ongoing training: Assess competency (eg, using mock codes).
  - Implement a QA/QI program to meet facility resuscitation standard.
  - Formulated response plan.
  - Continued staff development; keep up to date with current practices and stay safe.

Organizations providing hospital accreditation, such as the Joint Commission, require hospitals to collect data related to processes and outcomes of resuscitation and identify performance measures.

Early Defibrillation

Ventricular fibrillation (V-fib), a chaotic "quivering" of the heart caused by an abnormality in the heart's electrical conduction system, is the most common initial heart rhythm found in sudden cardiac arrest. Conversion of V-fib to a normal heart rhythm requires electrical defibrillation; CPR alone cannot correct it. Even with the most effective CPR, a person's chance of survival is poor unless he or she also receives early defibrillation. When defibrillation is delivered in the first minute following sudden cardiac arrest, the resuscitation rate can be as high as 90%. For every minute defibrillation is delayed, however, the victim's chance of survival decreases by approximately 7% to 10%.

Several states have legislated the use of AEDs by trained rescuers and bystanders. AEDs are now available even within hospitals. When applied to a patient in cardiac arrest, AEDs can reliably identify abnormal electrical heart rhythms (eg, V-fib) and advise the operator to administer a shock to correct the rhythm. Because AEDs are both simple to operate and economical, they could save hundreds of thousands of lives through early defibrillation.

Early Advanced Cardiac Life Support (ACLS)

Early ACLS is provided by paramedics in the prehospital setting and by other health care professionals including nurses and physicians in the hospital setting. ACLS includes advanced airway management, intravenous fluids, and cardiac medications to help stabilize the victim, as well as identification and treatment of underlying arrest causes, and preventing a recurrence of cardiac arrest.

If the patient survives cardiac arrest, he or she will need further advanced care to be able to return to his or her previous state of health. This may involve reperfusion (thrombolytic therapy), percutaneous coronary intervention (PCI)-stenting, and bypass strategies, as well as a team of specialists including physical and speech therapists, social workers, and family physicians working together to aid the patient.

▶ Legal and Ethical Considerations

Modern CPR techniques were advocated approximately 40 years ago. CPR instruction has become an accepted part of the health care system, in both medical and nonmedical settings. As litigation has increased, so has awareness of ethical and legal concerns involving CPR. Health care providers and rescuers need to understand these issues as well as their rights and responsibilities.

Duty to Act

What is the health care professional's **duty to act** to a patient? The duty of any health care provider is to have the knowledge ordinarily possessed and to exercise the care and skill ordinarily used in similar situations by trained and skilled members of the same profession in the same or similar circumstances. The duty as a health care professional therefore is to practice their profession as any other health care professional would.

The question still remains—when do health care professionals have a duty to act? Are you a health care professional 24 hours a day, whether you are working or not? Is it possible to form a health care professional–patient relationship beyond the scope of employment? The answer is, not necessarily.

Standard of Care

The quality of the care you provide to patients is based on training standards, laws, and authorities, such as national organizations, which guide your actions. This expected quality is commonly referred to as the **standard of care**. If you fail to perform according to this expected norm, legal action is likely.

Consent

A competent individual has the right to consent to, refuse, or limit medical treatment, even if this refusal might shorten a patient's life. A patient's right to choose among various treatment options (including no treatment) depends on his or her ability to give informed consent.

Because informed consent is impractical if a person is unconscious or otherwise unable to make a rational decision, the concept of implied consent is used. In these situations, it is assumed (implied) that the patient would consent to life-saving care if able to do so.

Advance Directives

Recently, efforts have been directed at allowing patients to make decisions before a crisis occurs. When informed decision making is done in advance of an emergency, it is popularly termed as an **advance directive**. Advance directives may include conversations, written directives, living wills, health care proxies, and durable powers of attorney for health care providers.

Although advance directives may be useful to you, their reliability and availability at the time of need may vary dramatically. You should familiarize yourself with the standards of practice and legal requirements in your area. A conversation with family, friends, or physicians is the most common form of advance directive. But conversational directives are also the most unreliable and easily challenged. Additionally, local practice statutes or regulations may define the acceptability of various forms of advance directives. You should be familiar with your facility or organization's directives.

Written advance directives are legally the most desirable forms of consent. To avoid confusion, a number of states and local health care systems have developed standard formats for advance directives in their regions. This standardized approach allows rescuers to identify and implement valid directives quickly.

Withholding or Discontinuing CPR

CPR is not always appropriate. The traditional contraindications to starting CPR were decapitation and clear signs of prolonged death, such as **rigor mortis** or dependent lividity. The indications to stop CPR were the rescuer's exhaustion; a direction to stop from a medical doctor; relief in duty by another, equally trained, person(s); or a situation that met the ILCOR Guidelines (Ethical Issues—Termination of Resuscitation). CPR should be stopped when no benefit can be expected because there has been no return of vital functions despite maximal ACLS therapy.

Currently, CPR can be withheld or discontinued if it is not desired by the patient, not in the patient's best interest, or not medically indicated. Some specific situations in which CPR may not be indicated include cardiac arrest due to trauma (injury) with an extended response time, situations in which your personal safety is threatened, and situations in which written protocols result in a decision that CPR should be withheld **Figure 1-8**.

Department of Health

Nonhospital Order Not to Resuscitate (DNR order)

Person's Name (Print)_____

Date of Birth ___ / ___ / ___

Do not resuscitate the person named above.

Person's Signature _____

Date ___ / ___ / ___

Physician's Signature _____

Print Name _____

License Number _____

Date ___ / ___ / ___

It is the responsibility of the physician to determine, at least every 90 days, whether this order continues to be appropriate, and to indicate this by a note in the person's medical chart. The issuance of a new form is NOT required, and under the law this order should be considered valid unless it is known that it has been revoked. This order remains valid and must be followed, even if it has not been reviewed within the 90-day period.

Figure 1-8

Do not resuscitate (DNR) form.

Emotional Support to the Families

Despite our best efforts, resuscitation attempts may fail. The notification of family members of a death is an important component of the resuscitation. This should be done as compassionately as possible so that the family understands that BLS and ACLS efforts failed and that the patient has died. Avoid using expressions such as "passed on"; be direct and concise. The health care professional should consider additional resources such as clergy members, religious beliefs, cultural diversity, and practices of the family.

Additionally, some reports suggest that it may be beneficial for family members to be present during resuscitation attempts. Although these reports show it may be helpful to be present during resuscitation efforts, many family members will not request to be present unless asked by the health care professional. The health care professional and the resuscitation team need to be sensitive to the presence of family members in the room.

Good Samaritan Laws

Good Samaritan laws exist in all states. They provide immunity and minimize liability in situations where rescuers act in good faith, within the scope of their training, receive no compensation, and where no negligence exists. Because the precise wording of these laws varies from state to state, you must understand what protection the laws of your state afford you.

prep kit

▶ Ready for Review

- As a health care provider, you are likely to be involved in the treatment of patients with cardiac emergencies. Your ability to provide these patients with the most appropriate basic life support is an essential skill. Although prevention remains critical to reducing cardiac incidents, emergency cardiac care is essential in sustaining life once an incident does occur.
- Emergency cardiac care includes providing CPR and other emergency care procedures to cardiac and respiratory arrest victims at the scene or in a health care facility. The Chain of Survival—early access to care, early CPR, early defibrillation, and early advanced cardiac life support (ACLS)—includes steps essential for successful resuscitation.
- Except in very specific situations, health care providers are required to perform CPR and other basic life support (BLS) procedures. Advance directives are a form of informed consent, made prior to an emergency situation, that enable a person to indicate, verbally or in writing, that he or she does not want CPR performed. Unless you have a reliable advance directive or are able to determine through specific criteria that CPR would be futile for the victim or dangerous to yourself or others, you should initiate CPR.

▶ Vital Vocabulary

acquired immunodeficiency syndrome (AIDS) The result of a viral infection caused by the human immunodeficiency virus (HIV).

advance directive Written documentation that a competent patient uses to specify medical treatment should he or she become unable to make decisions; also called a living will.

Advanced Cardiac Life Support (ACLS) The use of advanced airway techniques, administration of intravenous fluids and cardiac medications to help stabilize the victim, as well as identification and treatment of underlying causes, and preventing a recurrence of cardiac arrest.

atherosclerosis A disease characterized by a thickening and destruction of the arterial walls, caused by fatty deposits within them; the arteries lose their ability to dilate and carry oxygen-enriched blood.

cardiopulmonary resuscitation (CPR) Method that combines rescue breathing and chest compressions to treat the victim of cardiac arrest.

cardiovascular disease (CVD) A spectrum of disease processes affecting the heart and circulatory system; the leading cause of death in the United States.

Chain of Survival The four-step concept—early access to emergency medical care, CPR, defibrillation, and advanced cardiac care—that can lead to a reduction in death from heart disease.

coronary heart disease (CHD) Presence of atherosclerosis in the coronary arteries plus the presence of symptoms as manifested by angina or a history of acute myocardial infarction (from the American Heart Association).

duty to act The job-defined, legal duty to provide care.

Good Samaritan laws Laws that protect an individual from legal liability for errors or omissions when providing emergency care, in good faith, to a suddenly ill or injured person.

hepatitis A viral infection of the liver.

human immunodeficiency virus (HIV) A virus that attacks white blood cells and destroys the body's ability to fight infection; AIDS results from HIV infection.

personal protective equipment (PPE) Equipment that allows you to protect yourself, according to body substance isolation standards, from potentially contagious body fluids or bloodborne or airborne diseases.

prep kit

rigor mortis Stiffening of the body; a definitive sign of death.

standard of care Care that a reasonable, prudent person would provide under the same or similar circumstances.

tuberculosis (TB) A disease affecting the respiratory system that is caused by bacteria that settles in the lungs.

standard precautions An infection control concept and practice that assumes all body fluids are potentially infectious; infections are dealt with by creating a barrier between the rescuer and the victim.

ventricular fibrillation (V-fib) A rapid, tremulous, and ineffectual contraction of the myocardium (the heart muscle), producing no cardiac output; cardiac arrest.

▶ Check Your Knowledge

1. All of the following are avoidable risk factors for cardiovascular disease (CVD) except:
   A. cigarette smoking.
   B. heredity and aging.
   C. high blood pressure.
   D. stress and obesity.

2. Even with the most effective CPR, a cardiac arrest victim's chance for survival is poor unless:
   A. interruptions are limited.
   B. he or she is transported to the hospital in less than 10 minutes.
   C. the dispatcher provides prearrival instructions.
   D. early care is provided by ACLS-trained personnel.

3. Which of the following diseases is transmitted by the airborne route?
   A. HIV
   B. Tuberculosis
   C. AIDS
   D. Hepatitis

4. Over half of the deaths associated with coronary heart disease (CHD) that occur in a nonhospital setting are caused by:
   A. stroke.
   B. heart attack.
   C. high blood pressure.
   D. sudden cardiac arrest.

Answers: 1. B; 2. A; 3. B; 4. D.

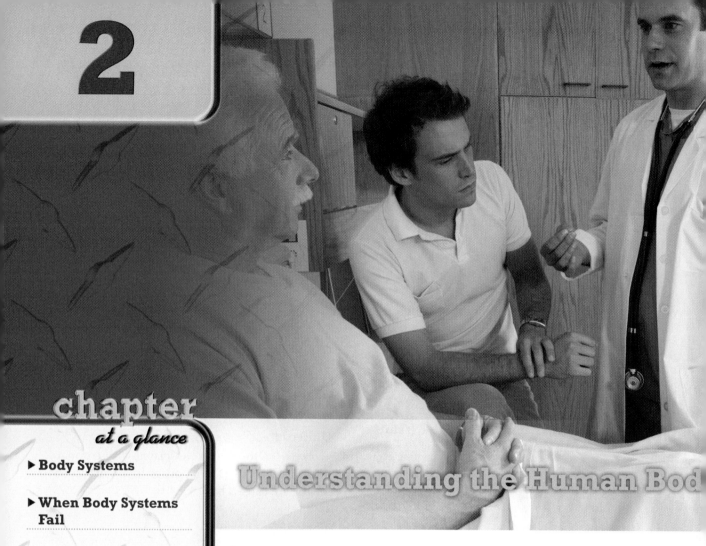

chapter
at a glance

Understanding the Human Body

▶ Body Systems

Failure of any body system causes serious medical conditions. The inability of one or more of these systems to function properly can lead to death. The challenge for the health care provider is to provide BLS to help sustain life and correct conditions resulting from the failure of these body systems—the nervous system, the respiratory system, and the circulatory system. This chapter provides a basic overview of these three body systems so that you can better understand their interrelationships when providing BLS care. For example, if the respiratory system fails, the nervous and circulatory systems will be deprived of oxygen. If the nervous system, specifically the brain, is without oxygen, the patient will lose consciousness. If the heart is without oxygen, it will fail to function. Similarly, failure of the circulatory system to circulate oxygen throughout the body will cause the other body systems to collapse.

The Nervous System

The nervous system is the command center of the human body. It is controlled by the brain, which regulates both the heart rate and the respiratory rate. The <u>nervous system</u> allows the body to react to internal and external stimulation, and the nervous system controls movement. Signals travel from the brain through a network of nerves that extend down the **spinal cord** and branch out through the body. These nerves act much like transistor circuits, sending and receiving messages at an incredible rate of speed (**Figure 2-1**).

Structure and Function

The brain and spinal cord serve as the headquarters and communication system for the body. They are well protected, because without them, all other systems would fail. The brain is encased in the skull, and the spinal cord is inside the vertebrae of the spine.

The spinal cord can be thought of as the main circuit board of a communication system. It relays sensory information from peripheral nerves to the brain and forwards signals from the brain to the body through motor fibers. Injury to any area of the spinal cord can disrupt the flow of information to and from the brain.

The brain has three main parts: the cerebrum (large portion of the brain), the cerebellum (small portion of the brain), and the brain stem (**Figure 2-2**). The **cerebrum** controls thought, sensation, memory, and voluntary motions such as walking or picking up an object. The **cerebellum** is located at the back of the head and below the cerebrum. It controls balance by coordinating signals from the eyes and inner ears. The **medulla oblongata**, located in the brain stem, connects the cerebrum and the cerebellum to the spinal cord. It controls involuntary motions, such as breathing, heart rate, and digestion.

Of all the organs and tissues in the body, the brain is particularly sensitive to oxygen deprivation. When either the respiratory or circulatory system fails, cells in the brain begin to die in as little as 4 to 6 minutes because of the lack of oxygen. Rescue breathing and CPR can help keep the brain oxygenated until the patient can receive specialized medical care.

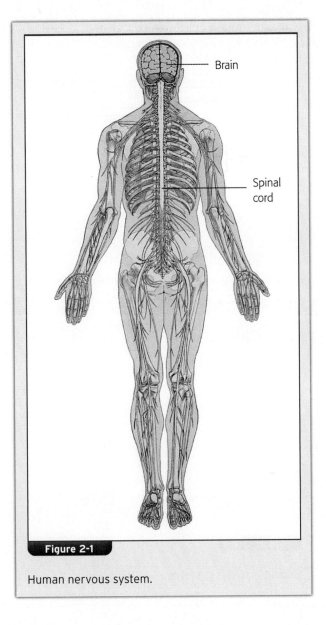

Figure 2-1

Human nervous system.

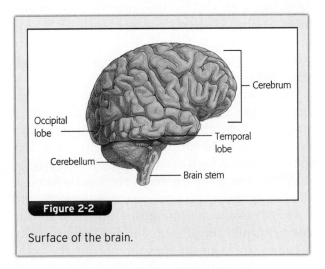

Figure 2-2

Surface of the brain.

It is important to determine, whenever possible, the patient's normal level of consciousness. For example, some patients may be awake, but unable to answer basic questions regarding orientation to person, place, or time. Knowing a patient's normal level of consciousness helps determine whether his or her current level of consciousness is a reliable indicator of injury or illness. When the brain is deprived of oxygen, the patient's level of consciousness can become altered. The alterations can be subtle signs in the beginning, such as restlessness.

The Respiratory System

Oxygen is the body's most vital external resource required to sustain life. The **respiratory system** delivers oxygen to the lungs and removes waste products such as carbon dioxide **Figure 2-3**. Because the body is unable to store oxygen for more than a few minutes, the respiratory system must function continuously. If it stops for any reason, such as in drowning or choking, the body will die within minutes.

Structure and Function

During respiration, air enters the mouth and nose, where it is warmed, filtered, and humidified. It passes through the **pharynx** (throat) and past the **epiglottis**, a small flap of tissue that lets air into the lungs as it keeps fluid and food out. Air enters the **trachea** (windpipe), which branches into two main passages called **bronchi** that enter each lung. Each bronchial tube divides into increasingly smaller tubes, ending in **alveoli** (air sacs) enclosed in tiny blood vessels called capillaries. The alveoli are where oxygen and carbon dioxide are exchanged **Figure 2-4**.

Air enters and is expelled from the lungs through the actions of the **intercostal muscles** (muscles of the chest wall) and the **diaphragm**, a dome-shaped, sheath-like muscle that separates the chest cavity from the abdomen. During **inhalation** (negative pressure draws air into the lungs), the diaphragm contracts (moves downward and flattens), as do the intercostal muscles. As the chest expands, the pressure inside the chest cavity becomes less than the pressure outside the body.

Air rushes in and expands the lungs to equalize the pressure. When the diaphragm and intercostal muscles relax, they force the air out (**exhalation**) **Figure 2-5 A, B**. Adults normally breathe 12 to 20 breaths per minute (respiratory rate). The normal respiratory rate for children is 15 to 30 breaths per minute; and the infant respiratory rate is 25 to 50 breaths per minute.

Normal respiration is an automatic process that occurs in response to the body's need for oxygen and the need to eliminate carbon dioxide.

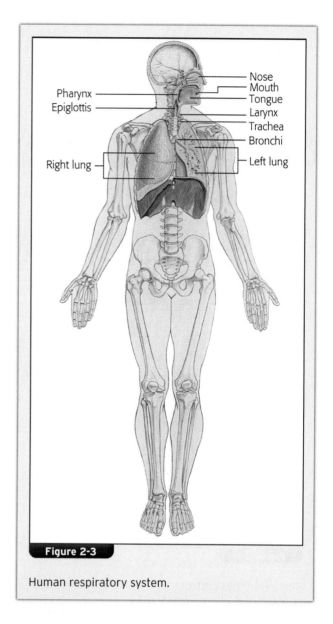

Figure 2-3

Human respiratory system.

Specialized areas of the brain sense the levels of oxygen and carbon dioxide in the blood and regulate the breathing rate and depth (deep, normal, or shallow) to maintain an appropriate balance of these gases.

The Circulatory System

The circulatory system is composed of the heart and the blood vessels. It functions to deliver oxygen and nutrients throughout the body and to remove carbon dioxide and other metabolic waste.

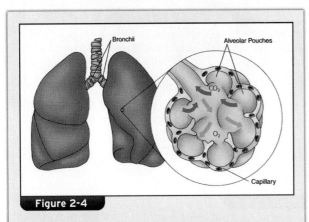

Figure 2-4

The exchange of carbon dioxide (CO_2) and oxygen (O_2) in the lungs.

Structure and Function

The **heart** is about the size of a person's fist. It lies behind and slightly to the left of the lower sternum, between the lungs and in front of the esophagus and the trachea. The heart muscle (**myocardium**) is essentially a dual-chamber pump with four chambers: the right and left **atria** and the right and left **ventricles**. The left and right sides of the heart are separated by a wall called the **septum**. The right side of the heart receives low-pressure, oxygen-poor venous blood from the body through the **vena cava**. This blood enters the right atrium and is pumped to the right ventricle and then to the lungs, where carbon dioxide in the blood is exchanged for oxygen. The oxygen-rich blood returns to the left atria of the heart, which pumps it to the left ventricle and then throughout the systemic circulation in the body **Figure 2-6 A, B**.

The heart (cardiac) muscle is unique among body tissues because it can generate its own electrical impulses without stimulation from nerves. This is called automaticity. In addition, the heart has special conduction tissue, which can rapidly transmit electrical impulses to the muscular tissue of the heart. The tissues that generate the electrical impulses are called **pacemaker cells** because they set the pace, or rate, for contraction of the heart. These pacemaker cells are located in nodes throughout the heart.

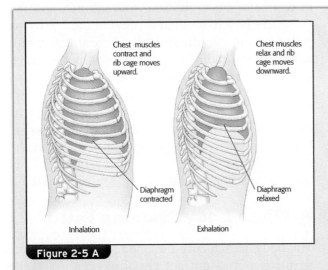

Figure 2-5 A

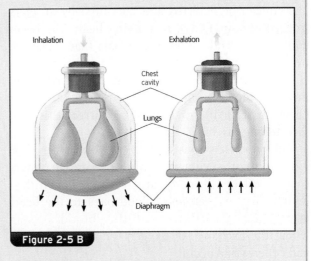

Figure 2-5 B

A. Chest muscle contractions. **B.** Inhalation and exhalation.

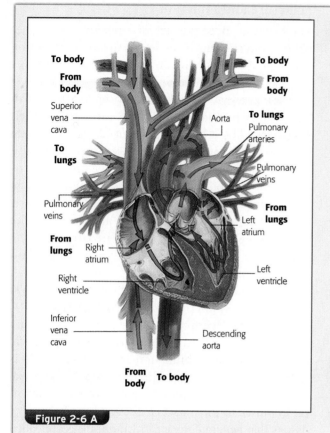

Figure 2-6 A

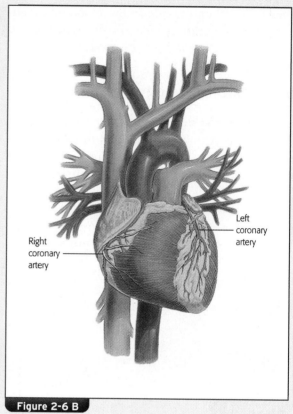

Figure 2-6 B

A. The heart in cross-section showing circulation, with arrows indicating direction of blood flow. **B.** An exterior view of the heart showing the coronary arteries.

The electrical impulses generated by the pacemakers can be detected and measured by an <u>electrocardiogram (ECG)</u>. In a dying heart, the pacemaker cells send out erratic signals that cause the heart to function irregularly. This produces a chaotic heart rhythm called <u>ventricular fibrillation</u>, in which blood is not adequately pumped from the heart. A <u>defibrillator</u> is used to correct this life-threatening rhythm.

Blood vessels consist of <u>arteries</u> and <u>arterioles</u>, which carry oxygenated blood from the heart to the rest of the body, and veins and venules, which carry oxygen-poor blood back to the heart **Figure 2-7** . <u>Capillaries</u> are tiny blood vessels where the exchange of oxygen for carbon dioxide and other waste occurs.

Each time the heart beats, blood circulates and a <u>pulse</u> is generated. The heart of the average adult at rest beats 60 to 80 times per minute, and the pulse can be felt at different areas of the body. The pulse felt on the thumb side of the inner wrist, alongside the radius bone, is known as the <u>radial pulse</u>. The pulse felt on the side of the neck, over the carotid artery, is known as the <u>carotid pulse</u>. The pulse felt on the inside of the upper thigh, at the femoral artery, is known as the <u>femoral pulse</u>. Check the pulse of an unconscious patient at the neck. Take an infant's pulse at the inside of the upper arm at the brachial artery (<u>brachial pulse</u>).

▶ When Body Systems Fail

The body, particularly the brain, lungs, and heart, requires a constant supply of oxygen. Without oxygen, cells in the brain begin to die in as little as 4 to 6 minutes. Without this critical command

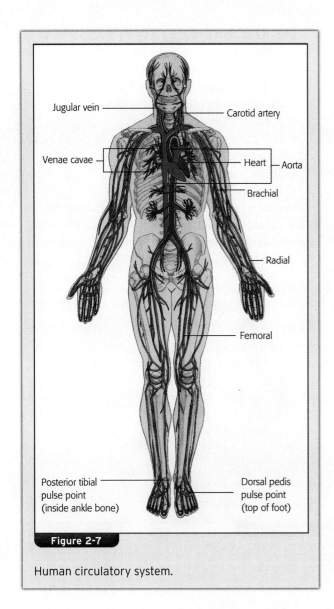

Jugular vein

Carotid artery

Venae cavae

Heart — Aorta

Brachial

Radial

Femoral

Posterior tibial
pulse point
(inside ankle bone)

Dorsal pedis
pulse point
(top of foot)

Figure 2-7

Human circulatory system.

the airway tissues to swell, narrowing or obstructing the airway. An airway obstruction can cut off the supply of air to the lungs.

The signs and symptoms of <u>respiratory distress</u> include:

- Signs of hypoxia, which may include restlessness, anxiety, and confusion.
- Signs of airway obstruction, which may include grunting, stridor, and an inability to speak.
- Flared nostrils.
- Tripod positioning.
- Unusually rapid, deep, or irregular breathing.
- Accessory muscle use (use of facial and neck muscles, retraction of muscles between the ribs, tracheal tugging)
- <u>Cyanosis</u> (blue color) of fingernails and around lips.

The most severe sign of respiratory system failure is <u>respiratory arrest</u>. In this condition, breathing stops and the skin becomes cyanotic or ashen. Without rapid intervention, brain cells die from oxygen deprivation.

Circulatory System Failure

Heart disease can narrow the primary blood vessels of the heart, the coronary arteries. When the inside of one of these arteries becomes so narrow that blood flow is restricted, oxygen delivery to the heart is diminished. This can impair heart function. A mild form of diminished blood flow can result in angina (chest pain).

<u>Angina</u> is a condition in which the heart is temporarily deprived of oxygen (<u>ischemia</u>) due to partial narrowing of a coronary artery. Angina usually does no permanent damage to the heart; however, it is a sign of heart disease, and persons with angina should seek medical attention. Angina is often brought on by strenuous physical exertion, stress, or extreme heat or cold. It seldom lasts more than 15 minutes and is usually relieved by rest and nitroglycerin tablets or spray, which dilate (open) the coronary arteries.

More severe or prolonged interruption of blood flow can result in <u>myocardial infarction</u> (heart attack). Angina and myocardial infarction are collectively referred to as acute coronary syndromes

center, the rest of the body cannot survive. The goals of CPR are to supply oxygen to the blood and to keep blood flowing to the brain until more advanced medical care is available. You should remember that the compressions of CPR produce a diminished blood flow and are approximately 30% as effective as the body's own functions.

Respiratory System Failure

Disease, injury, choking, drowning, or cardiac arrest can compromise respiratory status. For example, respiratory diseases such as asthma cause

(ACS). Signs and symptoms of ACS can include chest discomfort, fatigue, breathing difficulty, nausea, vomiting, and sweating.

Acute Myocardial Infarction

<u>Acute myocardial infarction (AMI)</u>, known more commonly as a heart attack, occurs when a portion of the heart muscle (myocardium) is deprived of oxygen to the extent that its cells begin to die (<u>necrosis</u>) **Figure 2-8 A, B**. AMI usually occurs as a result of atherosclerosis, a condition in which fatty deposits (plaque) significantly narrow or clog one or more of the coronary arteries **Figure 2-9 A, B**.

The signs and symptoms of AMI include:
- Chest pain or discomfort, radiating to the arms, jaw, or upper back.
- Difficulty breathing (dyspnea).
- Profuse sweating (diaphoresis).
- Nausea or vomiting.
- Irregular pulse in the presence of other signs and symptoms.
- Weakness.
- Cool, pale, moist skin.

Not all of these signs and symptoms are present in all cases. Approximately 20% of AMI victims experience no chest pain, a condition sometimes

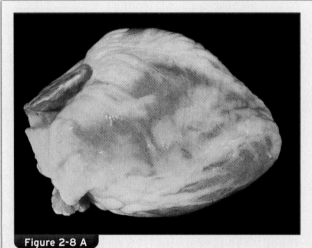
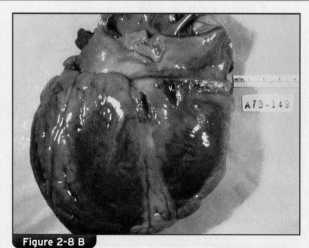

Figure 2-8 A   Figure 2-8 B

A. Healthy heart. **B.** Heart with artery clot after heart attack.

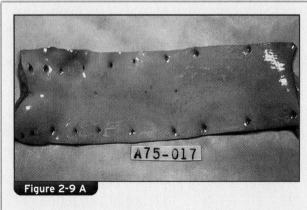
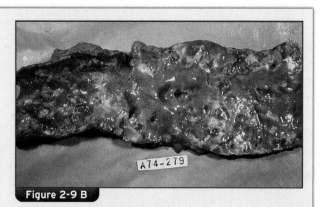

Figure 2-9 A   Figure 2-9 B

A. Normal artery (aorta). **B.** Atherosclerotic artery.

called a "silent" heart attack. Other patients—especially elderly, female, and diabetic patients—may experience vague or unusual symptoms such as weakness or "not feeling well."

The signs and symptoms of AMI are similar to that of angina, but are usually more intense. Chest pain associated with AMI lasts longer than 15 minutes and is usually unrelieved by rest or nitroglycerin. Patients with AMI are at risk for experiencing sudden cardiac arrest, especially within the first 4 hours after the onset of symptoms. The common pathophysiology is related to rupture of an atherosclerotic plaque. The ECG presentation may reveal ST segment elevation (STEMI). Effective interventions are extremely time-sensitive.

FYI

Many factors (pre-arrest conditions) are taken into account when making the decisions to withhold or continue resuscitation efforts. Currently, no consensus opinions exist. The pre-arrest morbidity (PAM) index, which examines the ability to predict CPR outcome, can be a useful tool to assist in making such a difficult decision. The PAM index is superior to using a single factor to predict survival after CPR in a hospitalized patient, but there is no clear consensus. It may assist in giving a practical basis for some difficult do not resuscitate (DNR) decisions. The patient variables used to determine differences in survival rates in the hospital setting include: age, gender, witness of the arrest and cardiac monitoring in effect, location of the event, advanced life support interventions in place at the time, reason for admission, previous cardiac arrest, pre-arrest functional capacity, and comorbid conditions. No simple, validated severity classification system is appropriate for all patients.

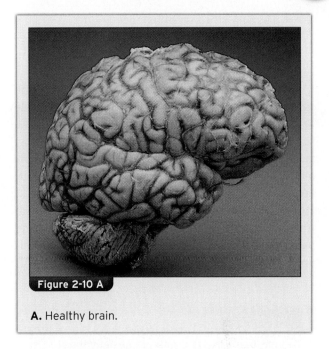

Figure 2-10 A

A. Healthy brain.

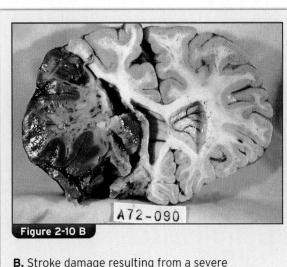

A72-090

Figure 2-10 B

B. Stroke damage resulting from a severe hemorrhage.

Stroke (Brain Attack)

Two types of <u>stroke</u> exist: ischemic and hemorrhagic. A stroke occurs when blood vessels delivering oxygen-rich blood to the brain rupture (hemorrhagic) or become clogged, so part of the brain does not receive the blood flow it requires (ischemic) **Figure 2-10 A, B** . Deprived of oxygen, nerve cells in the affected area of the brain cannot function and die within minutes. Because dead brain cells cannot be replaced, the devastating effects of a stroke are permanent. Strokes are the third leading cause of death.

The signs and symptoms of a stroke include:

- Weakness, numbness, or paralysis of the face, arm, or leg on one side of the body.
- Blurred or decreased vision, especially in one eye.
- Problems speaking or understanding.

- Dizziness or loss of balance.
- Sudden, severe, and unexplained headache.
- Deviation of the pupil of the eyes from normal.

Health care providers should use a stroke assessment tool, such as the Cincinnati Stroke Scale **Table 2-1** or the Los Angeles Prehospital Stroke Screen. These tools check for physical findings (eg, facial droop, arm weakness/drift, and speech abnormalities). Health care providers should also evaluate patients for other causes of altered mental status, including seizures and hypoglycemia. Although not every facility is capable of treating patients with acute stroke, plans should be developed for management of acute stroke patients.

Table 2-1 Cincinnati Stroke Scale

Test	Normal	Abnormal
Facial Droop (Ask patient to show teeth or smile.)	Both sides of face move equally well.	One side of face does not move as well as other.
Arm Drift (Ask patient to close eyes and hold both arms out with palms up.)	Both arms move the same, or both arms do not move.	One arm does not move, or one arm drifts down compared with the other side.
Speech (Ask patient to say, "The sky is blue in Cincinnati.")	Patient uses correct words with no slurring.	Patient slurs words, uses inappropriate words, or is unable to speak.

FYI

Cardiovascular (CV) disease is currently the number one cause of death in woman in the United States. Presentations may be atypical for CV disease. As a result, studies suggest that women are generally under-diagnosed and under-treated and have poorer outcomes.

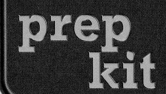

► Ready for Review

- The body systems that most concern health care providers are the:
  - Nervous system.
  - Respiratory system.
  - Circulatory system.
- The nervous system functions as the control and communications center for the body. The respiratory system supplies the body with oxygen and removes carbon dioxide. The circulatory system transports oxygenated blood from the lungs to the rest of the body. Each beat of the heart produces a pulse, which can be felt at various sites such as the inside of the wrist (radial), the neck (carotid), thigh (femoral) on an adult and child, and the inside of the upper arm (brachial) on an infant.
- The nervous, respiratory, and circulatory systems depend on one another for normal function. Respiratory system failure deprives the brain and heart of oxygen. Brain cells deprived of oxygen begin to die within 4 to 6 minutes and quickly become incapable of signaling the heart to beat.
- Oxygen deprivation to the heart can lead to chest pain (angina) or acute myocardial infarction (AMI), commonly known as a heart attack. Oxygen deprivation of the brain can result in loss of consciousness. A stroke occurs when blood vessels delivering oxygen-rich blood to the brain rupture or become blocked so that part of the brain does not get the necessary blood flow.

► Vital Vocabulary

acute myocardial infarction (AMI) Death of a portion of heart muscle caused by a coronary artery occlusion; also known as a heart attack.

alveoli Air sacs in the lungs where gas exchange takes place.

angina Chest pain felt when the heart does not receive enough oxygen.

arteries Blood vessels that carry blood away from the heart.

arterioles Smallest branches of an artery.

atria The two upper heart chambers that receive blood from the body and lungs.

brachial pulse Pulse found on the inside of the upper arm; used for checking pulse in infants.

bronchi Two main air passages that branch out from the trachea.

capillaries Small blood vessels that connect arterioles and venules and through whose walls various substances pass into and out of the narrow spaces between tissues and then on to the cells.

carotid pulse The pulse felt on one side of the neck, over the carotid artery.

cerebellum The part of the brain that coordinates body movements.

cerebrum The largest part of the brain, containing about 75% of the brain's total volume.

cyanosis A blueness of the skin due to insufficient oxygen in the blood.

defibrillator Device used to deliver a direct current (DC) shock to the heart to restore organized cardiac electrical activity.

diaphragm A dome-shaped, sheath-like muscle that separates the chest cavity from the abdomen.

electrocardiogram (ECG) Measurement of the electrical impulses generated by the cardiac pacemaker cells.

epiglottis The flaplike cartilaginous structure overhanging the superior entrance to the larynx and serving to prevent food from entering the larynx and trachea during swallowing.

exhalation The act of breathing out; expiration.

femoral pulse The pulse felt on the inside of the upper thigh.

heart The hollow muscular organ that receives blood from the veins, sends it through the lungs to be oxygenated, then pumps it to the body via the arteries.

prep kit

inhalation The drawing of air into the lungs; inspiration.

intercostal muscles Muscles between the ribs.

ischemia A lack of oxygen that deprives tissues of necessary nutrients, resulting from partial or complete blockage of blood flow; potentially reversible because permanent injury has not yet occurred.

medulla oblongata Part of the brain that is located in the brain stem and that connects the large and small brain to the spine; it controls involuntary functions, such as breathing, heart rate, and digestion.

myocardial infarction Death of a portion of heart muscle caused by a coronary artery occlusion; also known as a heart attack.

myocardium Heart muscle.

necrosis Death of tissues due to oxygen deprivation.

nervous system The brain, spinal cord, and nerve branches from the central, peripheral, and autonomic nervous systems.

pacemaker cells A mass of specialized muscle fibers of the heart that have the capacity to initiate an electrical impulse.

pharynx The portion of the airway between the nasal cavity and the larynx; the throat.

pulse The pressure wave that is felt with the expansion and contraction of an artery, consistent with the heartbeat.

radial pulse The pulse felt on the thumb side of the inner wrist, alongside the radius bone.

respiratory arrest The cessation of breathing; also called apnea.

respiratory distress A condition in which respiration becomes compromised from disease, injury, choking, or drowning; results in a limited supply of air to the lungs.

respiratory system The system of organs that controls the inspiration of oxygen and the expiration of carbon dioxide.

septum The wall separating the left and right sides of the heart.

spinal cord The cord of nerve tissue extending through the center of the spinal column.

stroke Occurs when blood vessels delivering oxygen-rich blood to the brain rupture or become clogged, so part of the brain does not receive the blood flow it requires; also known as a brain attack.

trachea The cartilaginous tube extending from the larynx to its division into the primary bronchi; the windpipe.

vena cava Two large veins through which blood flows from the systemic circulation into the right atrium.

ventricles The two lower chambers of the heart.

ventricular fibrillation Disorganized, ineffective twitching of the ventricles, resulting in no blood flow and a state of cardiac arrest.

▶ Check Your Knowledge

1. Acute myocardial infarction (AMI) differs from angina in that:
   A. AMI is the result of myocardial ischemia.
   B. chest pain caused by AMI often lasts longer than 15 minutes.
   C. nitroglycerin usually relieves chest pain caused by an AMI.
   D. AMI does not result in permanent damage to the heart.

2. The heart rate of the average adult at rest is:
   A. 30 to 50 beats/min.
   B. 40 to 60 beats/min.
   C. 60 to 80 beats/min.
   D. 80 to 100 beats/min.

3. Common signs of hypoxia include all of the following, except:
   A. anxiety.
   B. confusion.
   C. restlessness.
   D. flared nostrils.

Answers: 1. B; 2. B; 3. D; 4. A; 5. B.

4. A patient presents with sudden weakness, difficulty speaking, and paralysis to one side of the body. You should suspect:

    A. a stroke.

    B. angina.

    C. AMI.

    D. a silent heart attack.

5. Which of the following patients would most likely present with a "silent" heart attack?

    A. 50-year-old male with a history of hypertension

    B. 70-year-old female with a history of diabetes

    C. 45-year-old male who frequently abuses cocaine

    D. 62-year-old female with a prior history of a stroke

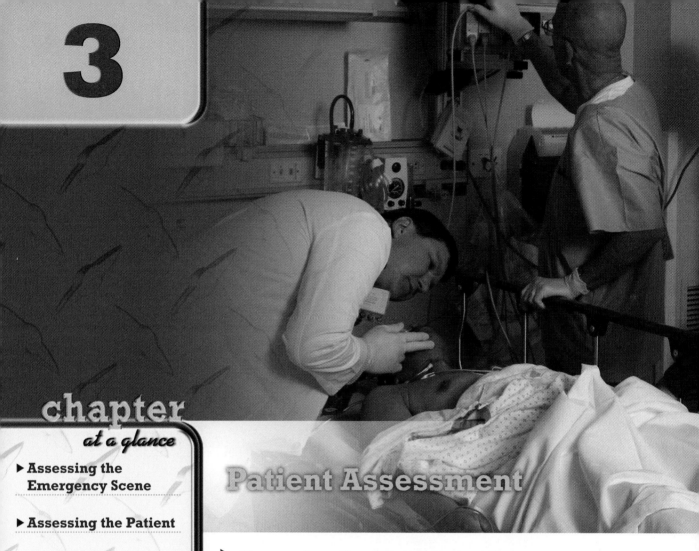

3

Patient Assessment

▶ Assessing the Emergency Scene

Your first task at the scene of an emergency (particularly out of hospital) is to quickly evaluate the area for hazards that could threaten the safety of those involved in patient care. This includes your personal safety, as well as the safety of other rescuers and bystanders. Your responsibility to assess the patient and provide care begins once the scene is safe ◀ Figure 3-1 ▶.

As you observe the scene, be aware of present and possible threats to safety. Scene assessment can also reveal possible causes of the patient's condition, from small, hard-to-notice items such as medication containers (possible medication overdose or nitroglycerin tablets for a heart patient) to more obvious causes such as near drowning or trauma.

Emergency scenes can be chaotic. There may be distraught family members and bystanders. Although these individuals can sometimes be helpful, they can also be a hindrance. There may also be many rescuers with different levels of training. If you are the person on the scene responsible for patient care, you must quickly gain control. Introduce yourself to other rescuers and bystanders in a calm and confident manner. Ask if you can help. Then determine whether the scene is safe and that you have adequate personnel and equipment to provide the necessary patient care.

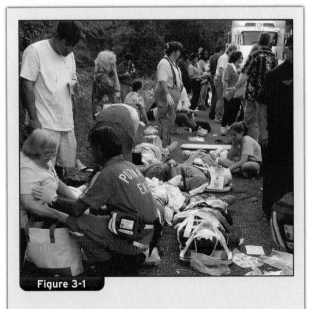

Figure 3-1

Assess patients and provide care once the scene is safe.

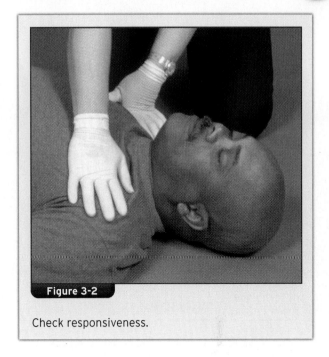

Figure 3-2

Check responsiveness.

▶ Assessing the Patient

Once you have sized up the scene and gained control, take standard precautions against disease transmission and begin assessing the patient. Effective care depends on accurate assessment. A logical, systematic format, known as the initial assessment, allows you to quickly examine the three most important body systems: nervous, respiratory, and circulatory. This will help you identify situations that present immediate threats to life.

Begin the assessment by checking for responsiveness (consciousness) **Figure 3-2** . If the patient is lying motionless, tap and gently shake his or her shoulder, and shout "Are you okay?" If the patient does not respond, he or she is unresponsive. This can indicate a life-threatening condition, which requires you to immediately assess the respiratory and circulatory systems.

Rapidly assess the respiratory and circulatory systems by examining the ABCs, answering five basic questions:

- Does the patient have an open airway?
- Can the patient maintain his or her own airway?
- Is the patient breathing?
- Is the breathing adequate?
- Does the patient have adequate circulation?

Airway

If the patient is responsive and talking, the airway is open (patent). If the patient is unresponsive, you must quickly search for the cause of the problem and attempt to correct it if possible. The first step is to open the airway. If you do not suspect a spinal injury, open the airway with the <u>head tilt–chin lift maneuver</u> **Figure 3-3** . This helps move the tongue away from the back of the throat and allows air to pass freely. If you do suspect a spinal injury, open the airway with the <u>jaw-thrust maneuver</u> without tilting the head **Figure 3-4** . It should be noted, however, that if the jaw-thrust maneuver does not adequately open the patient's airway, you should carefully perform a head tilt–chin lift. In some situations, simply opening the airway will enable the patient to start breathing on his or her own. These skills are covered in depth in the next chapter.

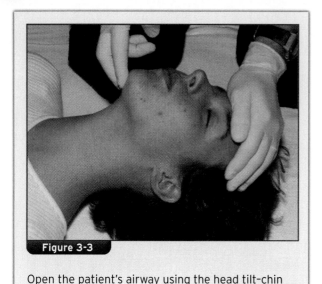

Figure 3-3

Open the patient's airway using the head tilt-chin lift technique.

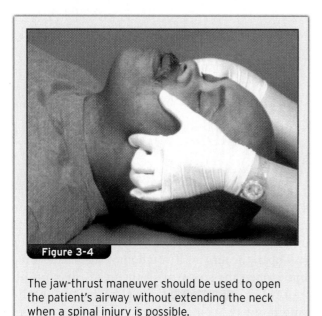

Figure 3-4

The jaw-thrust maneuver should be used to open the patient's airway without extending the neck when a spinal injury is possible.

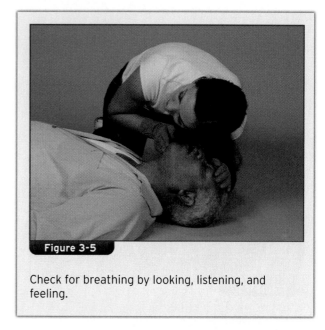

Figure 3-5

Check for breathing by looking, listening, and feeling.

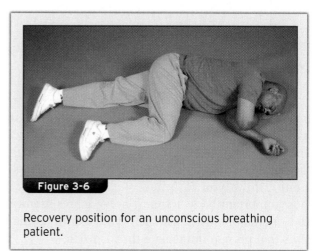

Figure 3-6

Recovery position for an unconscious breathing patient.

Breathing

Once the airway is open, assess the patient's breathing for at least 5 seconds but no more than 10 seconds. Place your ear a few inches above the patient's face with your eyes toward the chest. Look, listen, and feel for any indications of breathing **Figure 3-5**. Look for the chest to rise and fall. Listen for sounds of air movement. Feel for any breath from the victim's nose and mouth against your face. If the patient is breathing adequately, place the patient on his or her side (<u>recovery position</u>) **Figure 3-6**. This will keep the airway open and allow any fluid or vomit to drain from the mouth. If the patient is not breathing, or is breathing inadequately (eg, gasping breaths, slow rate), you will need to breathe for the patient, a skill known as <u>**rescue breathing**</u>. You will also need to assess for circulation. These skills are covered in detail in the next chapter.

Circulation

Once the patient's airway is open and you have begun rescue breathing, assess the patient's circulation. The presence of a pulse indicates there is circulation. Additional signs of circulation include:

- Breathing.
- Coughing.
- Movement.
- Normal skin condition (temperature and color).
- Improved level of consciousness.

If you are checking the pulse of an unresponsive patient older than 1 year of age, place your fingers in the groove between the Adam's apple and the neck muscle on the side of the patient's neck nearest you, and feel for a pulse in the carotid artery **Figure 3-7**. Never try to feel the carotid pulse on both sides of the neck at the same time. This could block circulation to the brain. Avoid using your thumb when checking a pulse. For infants (birth to 1 year old) check the brachial pulse, located on the inside of the upper arm. If signs of circulation are present, but the victim is not breathing, perform rescue breathing. If you cannot feel a pulse, begin CPR until a defibrillator is available. The skill of CPR is covered in detail in the next chapter.

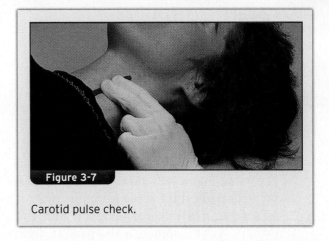

Figure 3-7

Carotid pulse check.

prep kit

▶ Ready for Review

- When you arrive at an emergency scene, you must first assess the area for potential safety hazards. If the scene is unsafe, make it as safe as possible for yourself and the patient. As you approach the patient, look for possible causes of illness or injury. Next, assess the patient by checking responsiveness and ABCs:
  - Airway.
  - Breathing.
  - Circulation.
- Open the airway and look, listen, and feel for breathing. If the patient is not breathing, you must breathe for him or her. Check for a pulse. If it is absent, begin CPR.

▶ Vital Vocabulary

head tilt–chin lift maneuver Combination of the two movements to open the airway in which the forehead is tilted back and the chin is lifted.

jaw-thrust maneuver A procedure for opening the airway in which the jaw is lifted and pulled forward to keep the tongue from falling back into the airway; maneuver used to open the airway in patients with a suspected spinal injury.

recovery position Position used to help maintain a clear airway in a patient with a decreased level of consciousness, no traumatic injuries, and adequate breathing.

rescue breathing The procedure in which a rescuer breathes for a patient who is unable to spontaneously do so on his or her own.

▶ Check Your Knowledge

1. What three body systems are examined during the initial assessment of a patient?
   A. Nervous, endocrine, respiratory
   B. Respiratory, circulatory, endocrine
   C. Nervous, respiratory, circulatory
   D. Circulatory, nervous, endocrine

2. The MOST important initial action to take on arriving at the scene of an emergency is to:
   A. call for additional assistance.
   B. determine if any hazards exist.
   C. immediately assess the patient.
   D. obtain information from bystanders.

3. When assessing circulation in a patient older than 1 year of age, you should:
   A. assess for a pulse at the carotid artery.
   B. attach an automated external defibrillator.
   C. lightly compress both arteries in the neck.
   D. assess for a pulse at the brachial artery.

4. Which of the following statements regarding the head tilt–chin lift maneuver is correct?
   A. It should be used to open the airway of non-trauma patients.
   B. The head tilt–chin lift maneuver prevents movement of the neck.
   C. Use this technique to open the airway if a spinal injury is possible.
   D. It takes two rescuers to perform the head tilt–chin lift maneuver.

5. The purpose of the recovery position is to:
   A. facilitate effective rescue breathing.
   B. protect the patient if a spinal injury is present.
   C. ensure the patient maintains adequate breathing.
   D. allow for fluid or vomit to drain from the mouth.

Answers: 1. C; 2. B; 3. A; 4. A; 5. D.

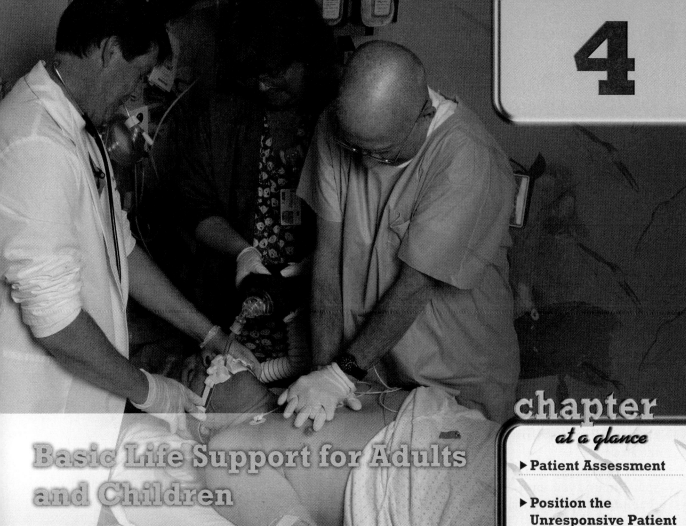

Basic Life Support for Adults and Children

▶ Patient Assessment

Begin every patient assessment by checking for responsiveness. Attempt to arouse a motionless patient by tapping him or her and shouting, "Are you okay?" If the patient is unresponsive (unconscious), check airway, breathing, and circulation. If no spinal injury is suspected, open the airway by tilting the head back and lifting the chin. Check for breathing. If the patient is not breathing, start rescue breathing immediately. If you cannot make the patient's chest rise during rescue breathing, the airway may not be adequately open. This could occur because the head is improperly positioned or because a foreign body is obstructing the airway. You need to correct this situation before rescue breathing can be effective. Once the airway is cleared and breaths go in, assess the patient's pulse. If there is no pulse, begin CPR by giving chest compressions and rescue breathing.

▶ Position the Unresponsive Patient

An <u>unresponsive</u> patient lying facedown needs to be turned onto his or her back. Roll the patient, keeping the head, neck, and shoulders aligned to avoid twisting the body and aggravating a spinal injury if one exists. Kneel at the patient's side and prepare to open the airway.

Open the Airway

When a person loses consciousness, all of the body's muscles relax, including the tongue. The relaxed tongue can fall back into the pharynx and block the airway. Because the tongue is attached to the base of the jaw, moving the jaw forward moves the tongue away from the back of the throat. Sometimes this is all that is needed to restore breathing. There are two common maneuvers for opening the airway: the head tilt–chin lift and the jaw-thrust.

The head tilt–chin lift maneuver is used when no spinal injury is suspected. Place one hand, palm down, on the patient's forehead and tilt the head back. Place two fingers of your other hand on the bony part of the patient's chin, and lift up **Figure 4-1** . This simple technique of opening the airway can sometimes restore breathing. In children, padding under the shoulders may be helpful. Take care not to hyperextend the neck as you tilt the head back; this could possibly cause the trachea to collapse or narrow, resulting in blockage of the airway.

If you suspect that the patient has suffered a spinal injury, you must open the airway in a way that protects the spinal cord. The jaw-thrust maneuver allows you to lift the patient's jaw without tilting the head back or extending the neck. Place your index and middle fingers on the angles of the lower jaw and your thumbs on the cheekbones. Move the lower jaw forward without tilting the head back. Because the patient will die if his or her airway is not open, carefully perform a head tilt–chin lift maneuver—even if you suspect a spinal injury—if the jaw-thrust is unsuccessful.

Check Breathing

Assess the patient's breathing for at least 5 seconds but no more than 10 seconds. While maintaining an open airway, place your ear a few inches above the patient's nose and mouth, and look at the patient's chest. Look, listen, and feel for breathing **Figure 4-2** . Look for the rise and fall of the chest. Listen for air moving in and out of the airway. Feel for air escaping on the side of your face.

Perform Rescue Breathing

If the patient is not breathing, rescue breathing is needed. Rescue breathing is the simple skill of blowing air into the nonbreathing (apneic) patient. Give the patient two initial breaths and then check

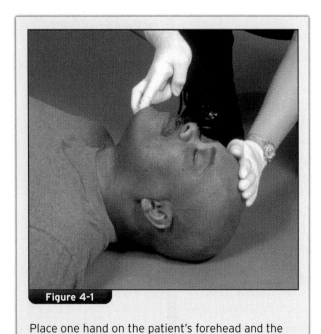

Figure 4-1

Place one hand on the patient's forehead and the other hand under the patient's chin.

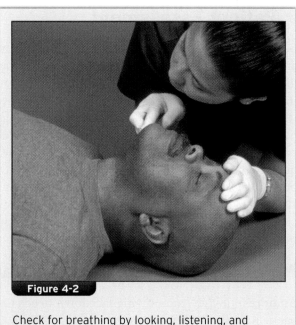

Figure 4-2

Check for breathing by looking, listening, and feeling.

for a pulse (signs of circulation). If the pulse is present but the patient is not breathing, you must continue to breathe for the patient. Rescue breathing rates for the child and adult are as follows:

- Child (1 year of age to onset of puberty [presence of growth of breasts in females and presence of underarm hair in males; approximately 12 to 14 years of age])
  - One breath every 3 to 5 seconds (12 to 20 breaths per minute)
- Adult (onset of puberty and older)
  - One breath every 5 to 6 seconds (10 to 12 breaths per minute)

Deliver each rescue breath over 1 second—just enough to produce visible chest rise. If it does not rise, reposition the head and try rescue breathing again. If this still does not work, suspect an airway obstruction that needs to be cleared. Treatment for an airway obstruction is presented later in this chapter.

Rescue breathing can be done with mouth-to-barrier ventilation devices, more advanced ventilation devices, or just your mouth. If you respond to an emergency, you should have the necessary ventilation or barrier devices to prevent disease transmission. When you are not on duty, you may not have ventilation devices readily available. In this situation, you must weigh the potential good to the patient against the limited chance of contracting an infectious disease through unprotected mouth-to-mouth breathing. To eliminate this risk, you should carry a pocket rescue mask or other barrier device in your car in case you need it when you are not working. Detailed information about ventilation devices can be found in Chapter 6.

There are several methods for performing rescue breathing, including:

- Mouth-to-mask.
- Mouth-to-mouth.
- Mouth-to-nose.
- Mouth-to-stoma.

Mouth-to-Mask Method

Follow these steps when performing mouth-to-mask rescue breathing:

1. Position yourself at the patient's head.
2. Open the patient's airway using either the head tilt–chin lift or the jaw-thrust maneuver **Figure 4-3** .

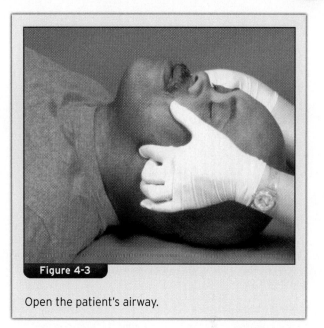

Figure 4-3

Open the patient's airway.

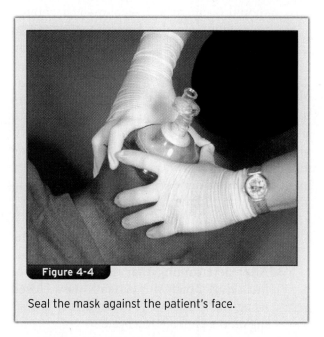

Figure 4-4

Seal the mask against the patient's face.

3. After determining that the patient is not breathing, place the mask over the patient's mouth and nose.
4. Using both hands, grasp the mask and the patient's jaw. Press down on the mask with your thumbs, as you lift up on the jaw with your fingers. This will create a good seal between the mask and the face **Figure 4-4** .

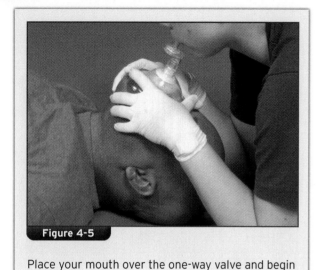

Figure 4-5

Place your mouth over the one-way valve and begin rescue breathing.

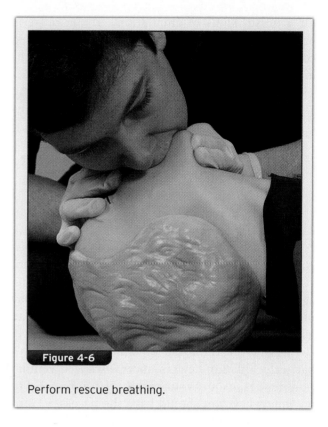

Figure 4-6

Perform rescue breathing.

5. Breathe into the one-way valve. Each breath should occur over 1 second—just enough to produce visible chest rise (Figure 4-5). Release pressure on the mask to allow air to escape.

Mouth-to-Mouth Method

Because there is no barrier in between your mouth and the patient's mouth, the mouth-to-mouth technique is the least preferred method for providing rescue breathing. However, if you do not have a mask or other barrier device, follow these steps to perform mouth-to-mouth rescue breathing:

1. Position yourself at the patient's head.
2. Open the patient's airway using either the head tilt–chin lift or the jaw-thrust maneuver.
3. After determining that the patient is not breathing, pinch the patient's nose closed using the fingers of your hand that is resting on the patient's forehead.
4. Make a tight seal by placing your mouth over the patient's mouth.
5. Give breaths as previously explained. Remove your mouth between breaths to allow air to escape (Figure 4-6).

Mouth-to-Nose Method

Certain complications necessitate breathing through the patient's nose, a method known as mouth-to-nose breathing. This is appropriate when you cannot open the patient's mouth, when you cannot make a good seal around the mouth, when the mouth is severely injured, or when the patient's mouth is too large or has no teeth. Mouth-to-nose rescue breathing is done like mouth-to-mouth breathing, except that you force the air through the patient's nose, as you hold the mouth closed. Open the mouth whenever possible to allow the air to escape (Figure 4-7).

Mouth-to-Stoma Method

A special situation involves a nonbreathing patient who has had a laryngectomy (surgical removal of the larynx). This patient no longer has a connection between the upper airway and the lungs. Instead, the patient breathes through a small, permanent opening in the front of the neck called a stoma (Figure 4-8). To check for breathing, keep the patient's head in a level (neutral) position. Place your ear over the stoma. If the patient is not breathing, perform mouth-to-stoma breathing. In some patients, there is still a connection between

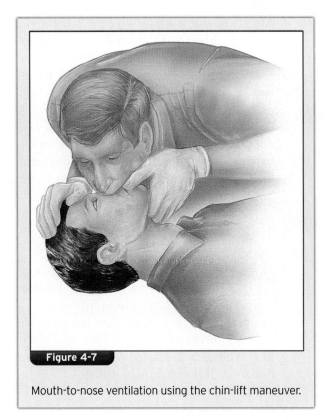

Figure 4-7

Mouth-to-nose ventilation using the chin-lift maneuver.

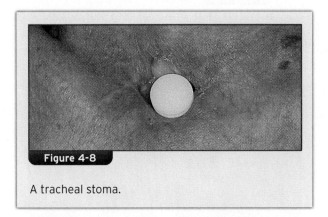

Figure 4-8

A tracheal stoma.

the upper airway and the stoma. When you breathe into the stoma, the patient's mouth and nose must be closed to prevent air from flowing into the upper airway.

Check Circulation

Once the airway is clear and your breaths produce visible chest rise, check circulation. Signs of poor circulation include pale, cool, or cyanotic skin; no movement; unconsciousness; or an absent pulse.

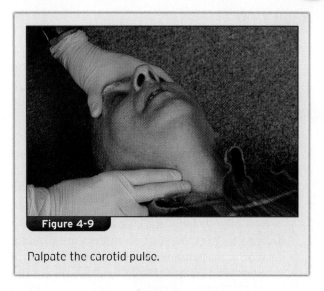

Figure 4-9

Palpate the carotid pulse.

In children, poor circulation is indicated by an absent pulse or a pulse rate of less than 60 beats per minute with signs of poor perfusion. Maintain the airway by keeping one hand on the patient's forehead (for the head tilt–chin lift maneuver) and use the index and middle fingers of your other hand to locate the patient's carotid pulse at the side of the neck nearest you. Locate the **thyroid cartilage** (Adam's apple)—the cartilaginous protuberance in the center of the neck—and slide your fingers toward you, into the groove at the side of the neck. Press down gently to feel for the carotid pulse. Feel for the pulse for at least 5 seconds but no more than 10 seconds **Figure 4-9** .

If the patient has a pulse, but is not breathing, continue rescue breathing. Recheck the pulse each minute to make sure it is still present. If the patient does not have a pulse (or the pulse is less than 60 beats per minute in a child with signs of poor perfusion), begin CPR.

▶ Perform CPR

CPR is a combination of chest compressions and rescue breaths. If the patient has no circulation, you must begin CPR and continue until a defibrillator is available. For patients older than 1 year of age, early defibrillation with either an AED or a manual defibrillator may be necessary to save the patient's life. Early defibrillation is presented in Chapter 6.

Adult CPR

Follow these steps to perform adult CPR:

1. Position the patient so he or she is flat on his or her back on a hard surface. Position yourself so that your knees are alongside the patient's chest.

2. Place the heel of one hand in the center of the chest, in between the nipples. Place your other hand on top of the first. Lock your fingers together and pull upward so that the only thing touching the patient's chest is the heel of your hand **Figure 4-10** .

3. Lean forward so your shoulders are directly over your hands and the patient's sternum. Keep your arms straight and compress the sternum 1½″ to 2″) using the weight of your body and not just your arms. Compressions should be fast and hard with minimal interruptions. Allow the chest to fully recoil between compressions. Give 30 compressions, counting each one out loud, "one and, two and, three and, four and, . . ." This will enable you to achieve at least 100 compressions per minute.

4. After 30 compressions, give the patient two effective breaths (1 second each). Ensure that each breath produces visible chest rise.

5. Continue the cycles of 30 compressions and two breaths for about 2 minutes (five cycles of CPR).

6. Recheck the pulse. If the pulse is still absent, continue CPR and reassess the patient every 2 minutes. If the pulse returns, check for breathing. If the patient is not breathing, perform rescue breathing.

Child CPR

Follow these steps to perform child CPR:

1. Position the patient so he or she is flat on his or her back on a hard surface. Position yourself so that your knees are alongside the patient's chest. Keep one hand on the patient's forehead, tilting it back slightly to keep the airway open, or place padding underneath the child's shoulders.

2. Place the heel of your other hand in the center of the chest, in between the nipples **Figure 4-11** . In larger children, it is recommended that you use two hands, as with the adult.

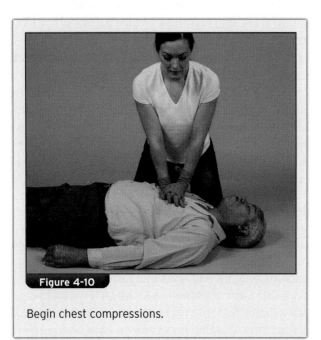

Figure 4-10

Begin chest compressions.

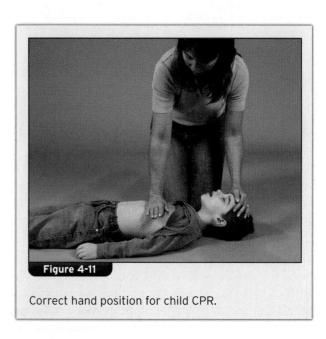

Figure 4-11

Correct hand position for child CPR.

3. Lean forward so your shoulders are directly over your hand and the patient's sternum. Keep your arms straight and compress the chest approximately one half to one third the depth of the chest. Relax between compressions, allowing the chest to fully recoil. Give 30 compressions, counting each one out loud, at a rate of 100 times per minute.

4. After 30 compressions, give the patient two effective breaths (1 second each).

5. After five cycles of CPR (about 2 minutes), recheck the pulse. If the pulse is still absent, continue CPR and recheck the patient in 2 minutes. If the pulse returns, check for breathing. If the patient is not breathing, perform rescue breathing.

FYI

When performing chest compressions, push hard and push fast. Provide 100 compressions per minute to a depth that is appropriate for the patient's age–1½″ to 2″ for the adult and one half to one third the depth of the chest in children. Allow the chest to *fully* recoil after each compression; doing so will maximize the amount of blood returned to the heart, and ultimately, the amount of blood pumped throughout the body. Limit interruptions in chest compressions to 10 seconds or less.

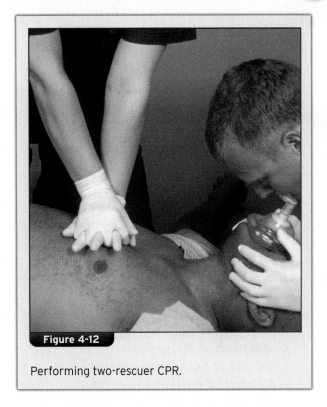

Figure 4-12

Performing two-rescuer CPR.

Two-Rescuer CPR

Whenever possible, two health care providers should work together to provide CPR. This has several distinct advantages over one-rescuer CPR:

- Rescuers do not tire as quickly and resuscitation efforts can be more effective.
- One rescuer can perform compressions while the other rescuer checks for the effectiveness of the compressions by periodically checking for a pulse. You should be able to feel a carotid pulse during adequately performed chest compressions.

In two-rescuer CPR, one rescuer provides chest compressions and the second rescuer provides breaths **Figure 4-12**. Rescuers should try to work on opposite sides of the patient, so they can switch functions without getting in each other's way. When you are performing two-rescuer child CPR, administer 15 compressions followed by two breaths. When two rescuers are providing CPR, they should switch functions after every five cycles (about 2 minutes) of CPR in order to minimize fatigue on the part of the health care provider. Unrecognized fatigue can result in chest compressions that are too shallow and/or too slow. The providers should switch positions quickly so that chest compressions are not interrupted for more than 5 seconds.

When an advanced airway (eg, LMA, Combitube, endotracheal [ET] tube) is in place during two-rescuer adult or child CPR, the rescuers should no longer deliver "cycles" of CPR. Instead, ventilate the adult or child at a rate of 8 to 10 breaths per minute (one breath every 6 to 8 seconds) and perform chest compressions at a rate of 100 per minute. Do not attempt to synchronize breaths and compressions; there should be no pause in chest compressions to deliver breaths when an advanced airway is securely in place.

Stopping CPR

You can discontinue CPR if:

- Return of spontaneous circulation (ROSC) occurs.
- Another trained rescuer replaces you.
- A physician determines it is OK to stop.
- You are too exhausted to continue.
- The scene becomes unsafe.
- Cardiac arrest lasts longer than 30 minutes, with or without CPR, except in cases of severe hypothermia or cold water drowning (according to the National Association of EMS Physicians).

CPR Complications and Errors

Even when CPR is done correctly, there are rare complications, including:

- Fractures of ribs and sternum.
- Separation of rib cartilage.
- Bruising of the heart and lungs.
- Puncture of the lungs, liver, spleen, or heart from fractured ribs.
- Ruptured lungs (pneumothorax; most often associated with excessive inflation of the lungs in children and infants).
- Gastric distention.

You can lessen the chance that the patient will experience these complications by paying careful attention to your "form." Do not let the situation make you careless. Some common mistakes people make in performing rescue breathing and CPR are:

- Failing to adequately open the airway.
- Failing to maintain an open airway once rescue breathing or CPR has begun.
- Failing to pinch the patient's nose closed or maintain an adequate seal over the nose and mouth.
- Not giving adequate breaths or breathing too fast or forcefully.
- Completing CPR cycles too slowly or too quickly.
- Failing to watch and listen for patient breathing.
- Not placing the patient on a hard or level surface for effective chest compressions.

- Doing chest compressions with the elbows bent instead of with straight arms.
- Performing chest compressions with the hands in the wrong location (often too low on the sternum, so that compressions are done over the xiphoid process).
- Using the wrong compression rate.
- Performing chest compressions that are too shallow, too deep, or with jerky movements.
- Not minimizing interruptions of CPR.
- Too many rhythm and pulse checks interrupt compressions.
- Breathing too fast or deep.

▶ Airway Obstruction

Airway obstruction (choking) is responsible for thousands of deaths each year in the United States. You must be able to quickly distinguish airway obstruction from other causes of sudden respiratory failure, such as a heart attack or stroke—conditions that require different treatment. Immediate recognition and removal of the obstruction is the key to preventing hypoxia (low oxygen levels in the blood), loss of consciousness, and cardiac arrest, which will ultimately occur if the obstruction is not removed.

Causes of Airway Obstruction

Food is the most common foreign body airway obstruction in a conscious adult. Small objects such as toys, coins, and pieces of burst balloon are common causes of airway obstruction in children. In any unconscious patient, the tongue is the most common cause of airway obstruction **Figure 4-13** .

Another cause of airway obstruction is swelling of the airway passages. Swelling can be the result of a variety of conditions, such as an allergic reaction, inhaling super-heated air (respiratory burns), croup, epiglottitis, or trauma. If you are unsure whether the obstruction is caused by a foreign body or by swelling, assume the obstruction is a foreign body. If you believe the cause of the obstruction is swelling, request advanced life support personnel.

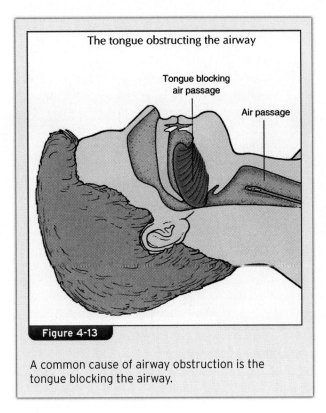

The tongue obstructing the airway

Tongue blocking
air passage

Air passage

Figure 4-13

A common cause of airway obstruction is the tongue blocking the airway.

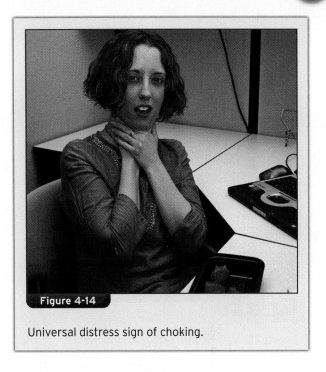

Figure 4-14

Universal distress sign of choking.

Types of Airway Obstruction

Airway obstructions are classified as being mild or severe. With a **mild airway obstruction**, the patient has good air exchange. He or she is responsive, can cough forcefully, and may be able to speak with difficulty. If the patient is coughing, encourage the patient to continue, as this will frequently clear the obstruction. Do not interfere with the patient's own attempts to expel the obstruction; this may result in a severe airway obstruction. Remain with the patient and be ready to intervene if the patient's condition deteriorates.

A **severe airway obstruction** occurs when the airway is totally blocked. In this case, the patient will be unable to speak, cough, cry, or breathe. The patient may display the universal distress signal for choking by clutching the neck with one or both hands **Figure 4-14** . When the airway is severely obstructed, the patient may turn blue (cyanosis) and will lose consciousness in minutes. Cardiac arrest will follow if the obstruction is not quickly removed.

Managing Airway Obstruction in Responsive Adults and Children

To determine whether a responsive (conscious) patient has an obstructed airway, see if he or she is able to talk and exchange air. Ask the patient "Are you choking?" If the patient nods yes and cannot talk, perform **abdominal thrusts**, also known as the **Heimlich maneuver**. This technique can force air from the lungs, creating an artificial cough that can expel the foreign object.

Follow these steps when performing abdominal thrusts on a responsive adult or child:

1. Stand or kneel behind the patient and wrap your arms around his or her waist. Tell the patient what you are going to do.
2. Make a fist with one hand and place the thumb side against the abdomen, just above the navel and well below the breastbone (sternum) **Figure 4-15** .
3. Grasp your fist with your other hand and give quick, inward and upward thrusts into the abdomen. The force of these thrusts will often be enough to relieve the obstruction **Figure 4-16** .

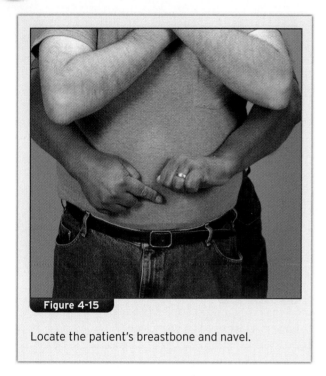

Figure 4-15

Locate the patient's breastbone and navel.

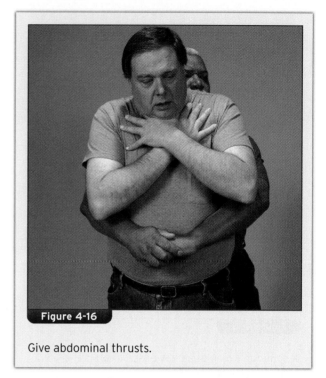

Figure 4-16

Give abdominal thrusts.

4. Continue delivering abdominal thrusts until the obstruction is relieved or the patient becomes unresponsive.

Special Situations

In some circumstances, you may not be able to reach around the waist of the responsive patient because he or she is obese. In females, the late stage of pregnancy may preclude you from reaching around the waist. Furthermore, you would not want to push on the abdomen of a patient in the late stage of pregnancy. In these situations, you can perform <u>chest thrusts</u> instead of abdominal thrusts **Figure 4-17** .

Follow these steps to perform chest thrusts:
1. Stand behind the patient with your arms under the patient's armpits and wrap your arms around the chest.
2. Place the thumb side of one hand in the middle of the chest, in between the nipples.
3. Grasp the fist with your other hand and pull inward on the chest until the obstruction is relieved or the patient becomes unresponsive.

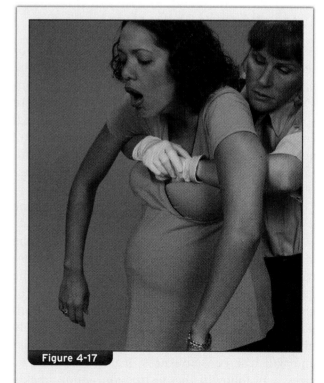

Figure 4-17

Give chest thrusts for a pregnant woman.

When necessary, you can perform chest thrusts on a supine patient by kneeling close to the patient and delivering downward thrusts in the middle of the chest, in between the nipples.

Managing Airway Obstruction in Unresponsive Adults and Children

You must assess all motionless patients in the same manner:

- Check responsiveness (consciousness).
- Open the airway.
- Check breathing, and if the patient is not breathing, provide two breaths.
- If the first breath does not produce visible chest rise, reposition the head and reattempt ventilations.
- If both breaths do not produce visible chest rise, an airway obstruction is likely.

Follow these steps when managing an airway obstruction in an unconscious adult or child:

1. Perform chest compressions, utilizing the same landmark as you did for CPR. Perform 30 compressions if you are alone or if the patient is an adult; perform 15 compressions if two rescuers are present and the patient is a child.
2. Open the airway and look in the mouth. If you see an object, attempt to remove it. If you do not see an object, attempt to ventilate.
3. If ventilation does not produce visible chest rise, reopen the airway and reattempt to ventilate.
4. If both breaths do not produce visible chest rise, perform chest compressions.
5. Repeat steps 2 through 4 until the obstruction is relieved.*

Once the obstruction is relieved and your breaths produce visible chest rise, check for a pulse. The patient may have been without oxygen long enough to cause cardiac arrest, which requires CPR.

*If you are alone with an unresponsive child with an airway obstruction, perform five cycles (about 2 minutes) of CPR and activate the EMS system.

prep kit

▶ Ready for Review

- Basic life support for adults and children follows the same general steps. Check responsiveness, airway, breathing, and circulation. Intervene at any point where the patient's airway is obstructed, the patient is not breathing, or the patient has no circulation.

- Use the jaw-thrust maneuver to open the airway if you suspect a spinal injury, and the head tilt–chin lift maneuver if you do not suspect a spinal injury. In children, take care not to hyperextend the neck. If the jaw-thrust maneuver is unsuccessful in opening the airway, carefully perform a head tilt–chin lift maneuver—even if a spinal injury is suspected.

- Rescue breathing can be performed by several methods: mouth-to-mask, mouth-to-mouth, mouth-to-nose, or mouth-to-stoma. Rescue breathing for adults should be performed at a rate of one breath every 5 to 6 seconds (10 to 12 breaths per minute) and one breath every 3 to 5 seconds (12 to 20 breaths per minute) for children. Avoid hyperinflating the lungs (hyperventilation), as this may result in an increase in pressure within the chest cavity and decrease the amount of blood that returns to the heart. Hyperventilation may also result in gastric distention. Be sure to deliver each rescue breath over a period of 1 second—just enough to produce visible chest rise.

- If the airway is obstructed in a conscious adult or child, kneel or stand behind the patient and perform the Heimlich maneuver. Give abdominal thrusts until the obstruction is relieved or the patient becomes unconscious. For an unconscious adult or child with an airway obstruction, perform chest compressions. Move to the head, open the airway, and look in the patient's mouth. Do not perform a finger sweep—regardless of the patient's age—unless you can see the object. Attempt rescue breathing again. If the airway is still obstructed, repeat chest compressions, visualization of the mouth, and ventilation attempts until the obstruction is relieved.

- If a patient does not have a pulse, or other signs of circulation, CPR is needed. CPR is a combination of chest compressions and rescue breathing. Chest compressions should be performed at a rate of 100 compressions per minute for adults and children. Perform 30 compressions and two breaths for adults and for all one-rescuer CPR. Perform 15 compressions and two breaths for two-rescuer child CPR.

▶ Vital Vocabulary

abdominal thrusts A method of dislodging food or other material from the throat of a conscious choking victim; also known as the Heimlich maneuver.

airway obstruction (choking) Airway blockage that prevents air from reaching a person's lungs.

chest thrusts Maneuver used to expel objects from conscious victims with an airway obstruction, particularly infants, obese patients, and pregnant patients.

croup An infectious disease of the upper respiratory system that may cause partial obstruction of the airway and is characterized by a barking cough.

epiglottitis Inflammation of the epiglottis.

Heimlich maneuver A method of dislodging food or other material from the throat of a conscious choking victim; also known as abdominal thrusts.

hypoxia Low oxygen content in the tissues.

laryngectomy Surgical removal (partial or total) of the larynx, usually due to cancer of the larynx.

larynx The organ of voice production; also called the voice box.

mild airway obstruction Condition in which the airway is partially blocked; the patient is able to exchange air in the lungs but has some degree of respiratory distress.

severe airway obstruction Condition in which the airway is completely blocked and no air exchange is possible.

stoma An opening in the front of the neck through which a person breathes if his or her larynx has been removed.

thyroid cartilage The cartilaginous protuberance in the center of the neck; also referred to as the Adam's apple.

unresponsive Without awareness; unconscious.

▶ Check Your Knowledge

1. An unresponsive patient is found lying face-down and does not appear to be breathing. What should you do first?
   A. Open the airway.
   B. Check for breathing.
   C. Roll him on his back.
   D. Check for a carotid pulse.

2. You attempt to open an injured patient's airway using the jaw-thrust maneuver but are unsuccessful. You should:
   A. carefully perform a head tilt–chin lift maneuver.
   B. hyperextend the head to ensure a patent airway.
   C. quickly place the patient in the recovery position.
   D. grasp the tongue and lower jaw and carefully lift.

3. A 6-year-old child has a pulse, but is unresponsive and not breathing. What is the appropriate rescue breathing rate for the child?
   A. 8 to 10 breaths/min
   B. 10 to 12 breaths/min
   C. 12 to 20 breaths/min
   D. 14 to 24 breaths/min

4. When performing rescue breathing on an adult or a child, you should:
   A. reposition the head if the first breath is successful.
   B. hyperventilate at a rate of 20 to 24 breaths/min.
   C. deliver each breath over a period of 1 to 2 seconds.
   D. ensure the chest visibly rises with each ventilation.

5. Proper treatment for a 5-year-old child who is not breathing and does not have a pulse includes:
   A. initiating CPR until a defibrillator is available.
   B. ventilating the child at a rate of 20 to 30 breaths per minute.
   C. compressing the sternum to a depth of 1½″ to 2″.
   D. performing 15 compressions and two breaths if you are alone.

6. It is appropriate to perform chest compressions on a patient with a pulse when:
   A. the adult patient does not respond to rescue breathing.
   B. the patient is responsive and has a severe airway obstruction.
   C. a child has a heart rate less than 60 beats/min and signs of poor perfusion.
   D. an adult has a heart rate less than 80 beats/min and signs of poor perfusion.

prep kit

7. When performing chest compressions on an adult or a child, you should place the heel of your hand:
   A. in the center of the chest, in between the nipples.
   B. on the lower half of the sternum, over the xiphoid process.
   C. on the upper part of the sternum, just above the nipple line.
   D. in the center of the chest, about 2″ below the nipples.

8. Which of the following is true of two-rescuer adult CPR in a patient without an advanced airway device in place?
   A. A compression to ventilation ratio of 15:2 should be delivered.
   B. There should be no pause in compressions to deliver ventilations.
   C. The ventilation rate should increase to 15 to 20 breaths/min.
   D. Rescuers should switch positions after every five cycles of CPR.

9. A 50-year-old male is unresponsive. You have attempted ventilation twice, but the chest did not visibly rise. You should next:
   A. perform a blind finger sweep of the mouth.
   B. open the airway and look in the patient's mouth.
   C. move to the chest and perform 30 chest compressions.
   D. reposition the patient's head and reattempt ventilations.

10. On which of the following patients should the rescuer perform abdominal thrusts?
   A. Responsive 30-year-old female who is 38 weeks pregnant
   B. Unresponsive 8-year-old child with an obstructed airway
   C. Responsive 19-year-old male who cannot speak or move air
   D. Unresponsive 5-year-old child who is cyanotic and not breathing

Answers: 1. C; 2. A; 3. C; 4. D; 5. A; 6. C; 7. A; 8. D; 9. C; 10. C.

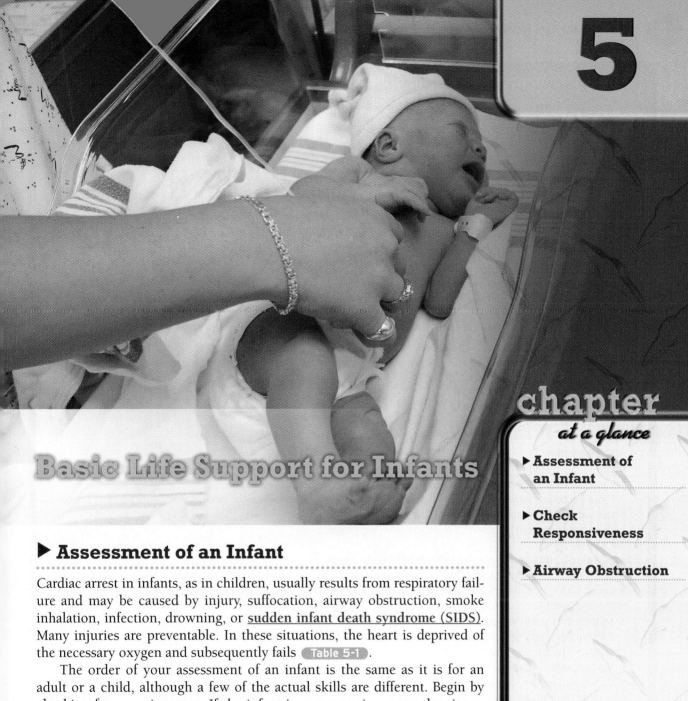

5

Basic Life Support for Infants

▶ Assessment of an Infant

Cardiac arrest in infants, as in children, usually results from respiratory failure and may be caused by injury, suffocation, airway obstruction, smoke inhalation, infection, drowning, or <u>sudden infant death syndrome (SIDS)</u>. Many injuries are preventable. In these situations, the heart is deprived of the necessary oxygen and subsequently fails Table 5-1 .

The order of your assessment of an infant is the same as it is for an adult or a child, although a few of the actual skills are different. Begin by checking for consciousness. If the infant is unresponsive, open the airway and check for breathing. If the infant is not breathing, provide the initial breaths. If the airway is obstructed, clear it so that air can pass. Check for a pulse. If a pulse is present, but the infant is not breathing, provide rescue breathing. If the pulse is absent, begin CPR.

▶ Check Responsiveness

When presented with a motionless infant, gently tap the infant and shout. You can also flick the soles of the infant's feet with your fingers to stimulate them. If there is no response, position the infant on his or her back and

Table 5-1 Common Problems in Children and Infants

Airway Obstruction
Mild Airway Obstruction:
- Good air exchange
- Child or infant is responsive
- Forceful cough
- Treatment: Allow position of comfort, assist young child to sit up (may sit on parent's lap); do not lay child or infant down

Severe Airway Obstruction:
- No crying or speaking
- Minimal or no air exchange
  - Cough is ineffective or absent
  - Increased breathing difficulty
  - High-pitched inhalation sound (**stridor**) or no noise at all
- Possible cyanosis
- Child or infant becomes unresponsive
- Treatment: Clear airway using the appropriate technique

Attempt Rescue Breathing
Sudden Infant Death Syndrome (SIDS) Signs and Symptoms:
- Sudden death in the first year of life
- Causes are not clearly understood
- Baby is most commonly discovered in the early morning

First Aid:
- ABC assessment
- Comfort, calm, and reassure the parents
- Try to resuscitate the baby unless he or she is stiff
- Parents will be in agony from emotional distress, remorse, and guilt; avoid any comments that might suggest blame
- Allow parents to be present during resuscitation attempt
- Allow parents to hold the child to start the grieving process

Child Abuse
Physical abuse and neglect are the two forms of **child abuse**:
- Abuse: improper or excessive action so as to injure or cause harm
- Neglect: giving insufficient attention or respect to someone who has a claim to that attention
  Signs and Symptoms of Abuse:
  - Multiple bruises in various stages of healing
  - Patterns of injury (eg, cigarette burns, whip marks, hand prints)
  - Fresh burns such as scalding, untreated burns, body part dipped
  - Parents seem inappropriately unconcerned
  - Conflicting explanations of injury
  Signs and Symptoms of Neglect:
  - Lack of adult supervision
  - Malnourished-appearing child
  - Unsafe living environment
  - Untreated soft-tissue injuries
  State Law Requires Reporting:
  - Report what you see and what you hear
    - Do not comment on what you think
    - Do not be judgmental
    - Do not accuse parents or guardians

attempt to open the airway. If you are alone, you should complete your assessment and provide 2 minutes of care before activating EMS. If two rescuers are present, one should activate EMS as the other cares for the infant. Remember that the majority of cardiac arrests in infants are caused by respiratory arrest.

Open the Airway

Use the head tilt–chin lift maneuver to open the airway of an infant unless you suspect spinal injury. Gently tilt the infant's head. The infant's head should be tilted back less than a child's. Be careful not to hyperextend the head and neck, which can collapse or close the trachea. To lift the chin, place your finger(s) just under it, on the bony portion of the jaw. Do not press on the soft tissue under the infant's chin, because this can interfere with opening the airway **Figure 5-1**. If you suspect a spinal injury, open the airway by using the jaw-thrust maneuver discussed in Chapter 4. Simply opening the airway may restore normal breathing.

Check Breathing

Take at least 5 seconds but no more than 10 seconds to look, listen, and feel for signs of breathing.

Look for visible movement of the chest. Listen for sounds of breathing by placing your ear next to the infant's mouth and nose **Figure 5-2**. Feel for air escaping from the infant's mouth or nose. If the infant is not breathing, you will need to provide rescue breathing.

Perform Rescue Breathing

If the infant is not breathing, create a seal over the infant's mouth and nose with a ventilation mask or with your own mouth, and give two slow puffs of air. Like the adult and child, rescue breaths for an infant require only the amount of air to produce visible chest rise. In the infant, this can usually be accomplished by providing ventilations with the amount of air that is in your mouth. As you gently blow into the infant's mouth and nose, watch for the chest to rise and fall.

If your breaths do not produce visible rise of the infant's chest, or if there is great resistance, the airway may not be completely open. Retilt the infant's head and try again. If the chest still does not visibly rise, the infant's airway is likely obstructed. Follow the procedure for choking described later in this chapter.

If breaths produce visible chest rise, check the infant's circulation. If a pulse is present but the infant is not breathing, continue to provide rescue

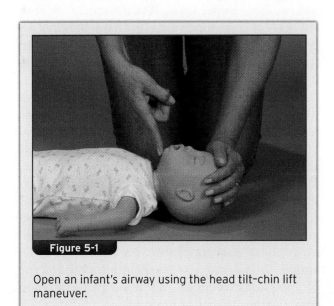

Figure 5-1

Open an infant's airway using the head tilt-chin lift maneuver.

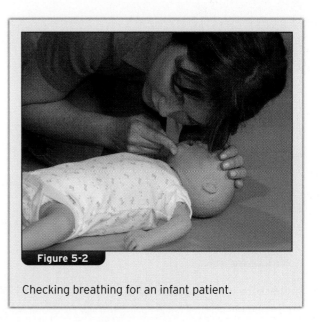

Figure 5-2

Checking breathing for an infant patient.

breathing. Because infants normally breathe faster than adults, you should breathe into an infant once every 3 to 5 seconds, or approximately 12 to 20 times per minute. Do not overinflate the infant's lungs by breathing too forcefully or too fast (hyperventilation). Hyperventilation can result in several negative effects; it may damage the infant's lungs, result in vomiting, distend the abdomen and make it difficult for the lungs to fully inflate, and decrease the amount of blood that returns to the heart. You can avoid these problems by maintaining an open airway and giving small puffs of air slowly (1 second each)—just enough to produce visible chest rise.

Check Circulation

Look for signs of circulation:
- Pulse.
- Breathing.
- Coughing.
- Movement.
- Normal skin condition (temperature and color).
- Improved level of consciousness.

Feeling the carotid pulse in an infant is difficult because infants have short necks. A better method is to feel the brachial pulse, found on the inside of the upper arm **Figure 5-3**. Place your index and middle fingers on the inside of the arm and press

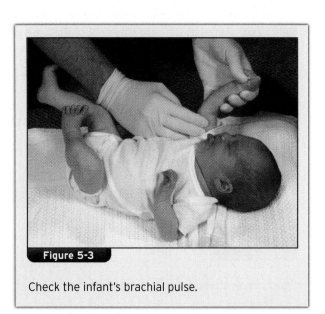

Figure 5-3

Check the infant's brachial pulse.

gently to feel the pulse. Feel for at least 5 seconds but no more than 10 seconds. If the pulse and other signs of circulation are present, but the infant is not breathing, provide rescue breathing. If there is no pulse, or if the pulse rate is less than 60 beats per minute with signs of poor perfusion (eg, poor skin color, unconscious), perform CPR.

CPR for Infants

CPR for infants only differs from CPR for adults and children because of the patient's size. Instead of using one or both hands to compress the chest, you use two fingers to perform compressions. Leave one hand on the forehead to keep the airway open. Place the fingers of your other hand on the infant's chest. To correctly position your fingers, imagine a line between the infant's nipples. Place your index finger along this imaginary line and your middle and ring fingers next to your index finger. Raise your index finger so that your middle and ring fingers remain in contact with the chest **Figure 5-4**.

With your fingers in the correct location, compress the chest with the pads of your fingertips. Compress the chest approximately one half to one third the depth of the chest, at a rate of 100 compressions per minute. Ensure that the chest fully recoils following each compression.

If you are by yourself, give 30 compressions and two breaths per cycle. If two rescuers are present, give 15 compressions and two breaths per cycle. As with adult and child CPR, two rescuers should switch roles every 2 minutes in order to minimize rescuer fatigue. Perform five cycles (about 2 minutes) of CPR, then recheck the pulse. If the pulse is still absent, continue CPR and recheck the pulse every 2 minutes thereafter.

When an advanced airway (eg, laryngeal mask airway [LMA], endotracheal [ET] tube) is in place during two-rescuer infant CPR, the rescuers should no longer deliver "cycles" of CPR. Instead, ventilate the infant at a rate of 8 to 10 breaths per minute (one breath every 6 to 8 seconds) and perform chest compressions at a rate of 100 per minute. Do not attempt to synchronize breaths and compressions; there should be no pause in chest compressions to deliver breaths.

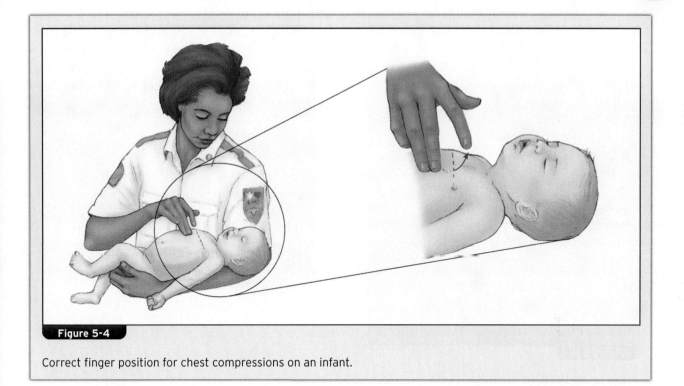

Figure 5-4

Correct finger position for chest compressions on an infant.

FYI

When two rescuers are performing CPR on an infant, the two-thumb technique should be used, with the hands encircling the infant's chest **Figure 5-5** . This method has been shown to provide better blood flow than the two-finger method and is less tiresome for the rescuer performing compressions.

Figure 5-5
The two-thumb technique is the primary method of providing chest compressions to the infant when there are two rescuers.

▶ Airway Obstruction

Managing the Responsive Infant With an Airway Obstruction

Like children, infants also choke on food such as meat, grapes, and nuts and small objects such as toys, coins, and pieces of burst balloon. An infant who exhibits signs of choking or one who is coughing may have an airway obstruction. If the infant is coughing forcefully, has good air exchange, and normal skin color, suspect a mild airway obstruction. Closely observe the infant, but do not interfere with his or her own attempts to expel the obstruction. If the infant cannot cough, cry, or breathe, is coughing weakly, turning blue (cyanosis), or making high-pitched sounds during inhalation (stridor), he or she has a severe airway obstruction and requires your immediate assistance.

Follow these steps to provide care for a conscious infant with a severe airway obstruction:

1. Position the infant facedown over your forearm with his or her head lower than the chest. Support the infant's jaw with your hand.

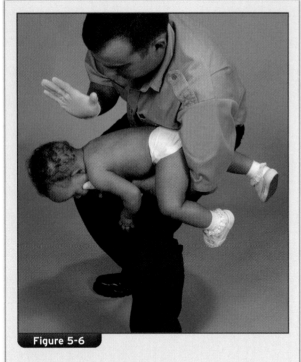

Figure 5-6

Correct position for administering back slaps to an infant.

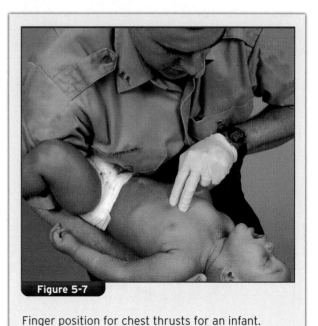

Figure 5-7

Finger position for chest thrusts for an infant.

2. Lower the infant and your forearm to your thigh.
3. Use the heel of your hand to give the infant five back slaps between the shoulder blades **Figure 5-6** . Deliver each slap with enough force to dislodge the obstruction.
4. Place the infant between your hands and arms and turn the infant face up.
5. If the back slaps did not dislodge the foreign body, give five chest thrusts. Place three fingers on the sternum, with your ring finger on an imaginary line connecting the infant's nipples. Lift your index finger and give five distinct thrusts with your ring and middle fingers on the sternum **Figure 5-7** .
6. Observe the infant throughout the process to see whether the obstruction has been cleared. If it has not, continue the cycles of five back slaps and five chest thrusts until the obstruction is cleared or the infant becomes unconscious.

Managing the Unresponsive Infant With an Airway Obstruction

When you are presented with a motionless infant, check the infant for responsiveness. If the infant is unresponsive, position the infant on his or her back on a firm surface. Open the airway using the head tilt–chin lift maneuver. Look, listen, and feel for breathing for at least 5 seconds but no more than 10 seconds. If breathing is absent, attempt to give a breath. If the chest does not visibly rise, reposition the infant's head and try again. If the second attempt fails, the airway is likely obstructed and requires immediate treatment.

Follow these steps when managing an airway obstruction in an unconscious infant:

1. Position the infant on a firm, flat surface.
2. Open the infant's airway and look for an object in the mouth **Figure 5-8** . If the object is visible, remove it. Do not perform a blind finger sweep.
3. Attempt to ventilate. If unsuccessful, reposition the infant's head and reattempt to ventilate.

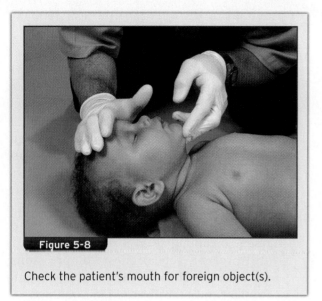

Figure 5-8

Check the patient's mouth for foreign object(s).

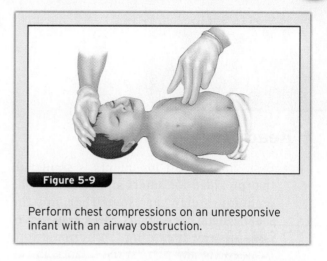

Figure 5-9

Perform chest compressions on an unresponsive infant with an airway obstruction.

4. If both breaths do not produce visible chest rise, begin chest compressions using the same landmark previously discussed Figure 5-9 . If you are alone, perform 30 compressions. If two rescuers are present, perform 15 chest compressions.

5. Repeat steps 2 through 4 until the obstruction is removed. After five cycles (about 2 minutes) of CPR, activate the EMS system.

prep kit

▶ Ready for Review

- Basic life support for infants is similar to that provided for adults and children. The techniques may vary somewhat, but the same general steps apply: check responsiveness, airway, breathing, and circulation. Intervene at any point if the infant's airway is obstructed, if the infant is not breathing, if the infant is pulseless, or if the infant has a heart rate less than 60 beats per minute with signs of poor perfusion.

- Open the infant's airway by using the head tilt–chin lift maneuver if you do not suspect a spinal injury. Be careful not to hyperextend the neck; this could cause the trachea to collapse or narrow. If the infant is not breathing, provide two initial breaths. If these breaths produce visible chest rise, check for a brachial pulse. If there is a pulse, but the infant is not breathing, continue rescue breathing by giving one small breath (1 second each) every 3 to 5 seconds. Recheck the pulse each minute.

- If there is no pulse, or if the pulse rate is less than 60 beats per minute with poor perfusion, begin CPR. If you are alone, use two fingers to compress the chest 30 times, at a rate of 100 compressions per minute, to a depth equal to one half to one third the depth of the chest. After 30 compressions, give two breaths. If two rescuers are present, use the two-thumb technique with the hands encircling the chest and provide 15 compressions to two breaths. Continue CPR for five cycles (about 2 minutes) and then recheck the pulse. If the pulse is still absent, or less than 60 beats per minute with poor perfusion, continue CPR. If the pulse returns (or increases above 60 beats per minute), but the infant is still not breathing, provide rescue breathing.

- If your breath does not produce visible chest rise, reposition the head and try again. If both breaths do not produce visible chest rise, the airway is obstructed. Place the infant on a hard, flat surface and begin chest compressions (30 compressions if you are alone, 15 compressions if two rescuers are present). After chest compressions, open the infant's airway and look in the mouth. Remove the object only if you can see it; do not perform a blind finger sweep. Attempt rescue breathing again. If the obstruction is still present, repeat chest compressions, visualization of the mouth, and attempts to ventilate until the obstruction is relieved.

▶ Vital Vocabulary

child abuse Any improper or excessive action that injures or otherwise harms a child or infant; includes neglect and physical, sexual, and emotional abuse.

stridor High-pitched sound heard during inhalation; indicates obstruction of the upper airway.

sudden infant death syndrome (SIDS) Death of an infant or young child that remains unexplained after a complete autopsy.

▶ Check Your Knowledge

1. After determining that an infant is unresponsive, you should:
   A. hyperextend the neck to open the airway.
   B. gently lift the chin and tilt the head back.
   C. look, listen, and feel for signs of breathing.
   D. perform CPR for 2 minutes and then reassess.

2. If you are alone with an infant who is not breathing and does not have a pulse, you should deliver a compression to ventilation ratio of:
   A. 5:1.
   B. 15:2.
   C. 30:2.
   D. 50:2.

3. In which of the following situations should you perform CPR on an infant?

A. Not breathing, brachial pulse rate of 90 beats/min, and cyanosis

B. Slow breathing, brachial pulse rate of 100 beats/min, pink skin

C. Slow breathing, brachial pulse rate of 80 beats/min, cyanosis

D. Not breathing, brachial pulse rate of 50 beats/min, cyanosis

4. During two-rescuer infant CPR, chest compressions should be performed:

A. at a rate of 80 to 100 per minute to a depth of 1½″ to 2″.

B. with two fingers over the sternum, just below the nipple line.

C. with two thumbs and the hands encircling the infant's chest.

D. by allowing partial recoil of the chest before compressing again.

5. Which of the following represents the correct sequence for managing an unresponsive infant with a severe airway obstruction?

A. Chest compressions, visualize the mouth, attempt to ventilate

B. Abdominal thrusts, finger sweep of the mouth, attempt to ventilate

C. Chest compressions, back slaps, visualize the mouth, attempt to ventilate

D. Back slaps, chest thrusts, finger sweep of the mouth, attempt to ventilate

6. You and your partner are performing CPR on a 6-month-old infant. At what point should you and your partner switch positions?

A. After 10 cycles (about 4 minutes) of CPR

B. When you become physically fatigued

C. After 2 minutes (five cycles) of CPR

D. After an advanced airway is placed

7. Ventilating an infant with breaths that are too fast or too forceful will most likely result in:

A. increased blood return to the heart.

B. decreased blood return to the heart.

C. too much oxygen in the infant's blood.

D. underinflation of the infant's lungs.

Answers: 1. B; 2. C; 3. D; 4. C; 5. A; 6. C; 7. B.

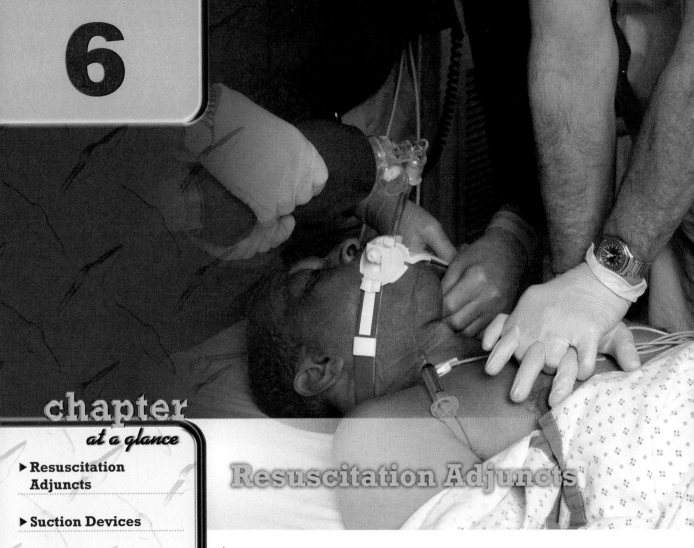

6

chapter *at a glance*

Resuscitation Adjuncts

▶ Resuscitation Adjuncts

Successfully managing respiratory and cardiac emergencies requires quick thinking, sound skills, teamwork, and familiarity with how your equipment operates. When correctly used, suction units help clear the airway, airway devices help maintain an open airway, ventilation devices provide effective barriers against disease transmission, and defibrillators enhance the chance of survival for cardiac arrest patients.

▶ Suction Devices

Patients who have vomited, inhaled fluid or debris, are unable to maintain their own airway, or who are bleeding from the nose or mouth are in danger of an airway obstruction. You cannot maintain an open airway or begin rescue breathing until the airway is clear and effective air exchange can occur. Suction devices can help you remove secretions from the airway, thus preventing them from obstructing the airway or being inhaled into the trachea and lungs (aspiration). There are two primary types of suction devices: manual devices and mechanical devices.

Manual Suction Devices

Manual suction devices that do not require batteries or an electrical source are among the most convenient to operate. These devices are always ready to work and require minimal servicing. Suction is applied by inserting the tip of the device into the patient's mouth and squeezing its handle to create a vacuum that withdraws debris **Figure 6-1**. Manual and mechanical suction devices are used in the same way, described in detail in the following section; the only difference is the power source.

Mechanical Suction Devices

Mechanical suction units are powered by rechargeable batteries, pressurized oxygen, or pneumatic (vacuum) devices. These units require familiarity with the mechanisms for their use, as well as regular maintenance and service checks **Figure 6-2**. Like manual suction devices, these mechanical devices also create a vacuum that draws obstructing materials from the patient's airway. To use these devices effectively, you must learn how they operate and how to control the force of the suction.

All mechanical suction devices consist of a power unit, disposable suction catheters of various sizes and shapes, an unbreakable collection bottle, suction tubing, and a supply of water for flushing out the tubing and suction catheters. Two types of suction tips are commonly used with mechanical

suction devices: the rigid-tip catheter **Figure 6-3** and the flexible whistle-tip catheter **Figure 6-4**.

Follow these steps when suctioning:

1. Turn the patient's head to the side. If you suspect a spinal injury, roll the patient onto his or her side and keep the neck and body from twisting.
2. Open the patient's mouth and wipe away any large debris with your gloved fingers.
3. Measure the suction catheter from the corner of the patient's mouth to the earlobe. This gives you the proper depth to insert

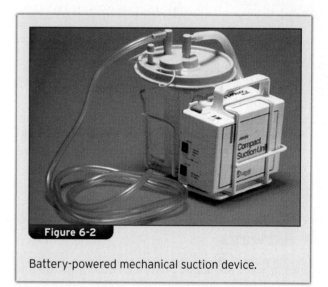

Figure 6-2

Battery-powered mechanical suction device.

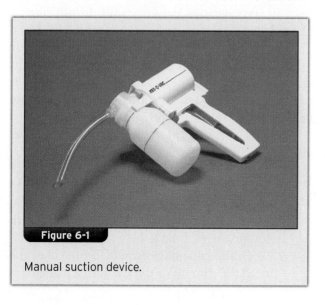

Figure 6-1

Manual suction device.

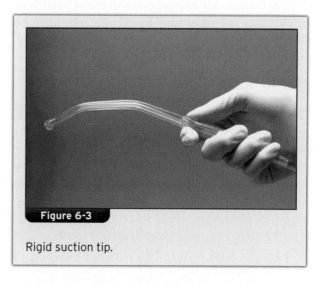

Figure 6-3

Rigid suction tip.

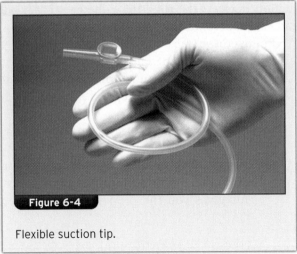

Figure 6-4

Flexible suction tip.

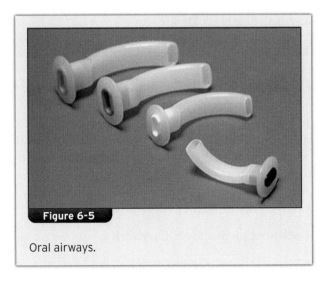

Figure 6-5

Oral airways.

the end of the suction tip. Inserting the catheter too deeply and attempting to suction is likely to stimulate the patient's vomiting (gag) reflex.

4. Turn on the suction device, insert the suction tip, and suction as you slowly withdraw the catheter from the mouth. In adults, suction for no longer than 15 seconds (10 seconds in children and 5 seconds in infants).

▶ Airways

Once a patient's airway is clear, maintaining the open airway is extremely important. Because the tongue is the most common cause of airway obstruction in an unconscious patient, artificial airways can be used to prevent the tongue from blocking the airway. There are two types of airways: oral and nasal.

Oral Airways

The most commonly used airway is the <u>oropharyngeal (oral) airway</u> **Figure 6-5**. It is inserted along the roof of the mouth and rotated into position in the back of the throat. The flange end rests on the lips. This position keeps the tongue from falling back into the throat and obstructing the airway. Improper placement could force the tongue farther into the pharynx, resulting in airway obstruction. Because the oral airway will likely stimulate the

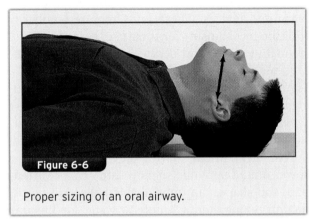

Figure 6-6

Proper sizing of an oral airway.

oropharynx and cause gagging, it should only be used in unconscious patients who do not have a gag reflex.

There are various sizes of oral airways for infants, children, and adults. Selecting the right size is important. If the oral airway is too large, it can trigger the gag reflex, and vomit could possibly be aspirated into the trachea and lungs.

Follow these steps when inserting an oral airway:

1. Choose the right size. Measure the device from the corner of the patient's mouth to the earlobe **Figure 6-6**. Alternatively, you can measure from the corner of the mouth to the angle of the jaw.

2. Open the patient's airway by using either the head tilt-chin lift or the jaw-thrust maneuver.

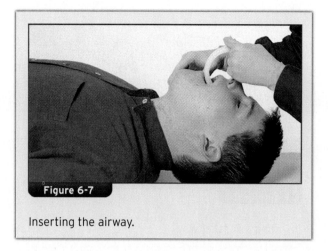

Figure 6-7

Inserting the airway.

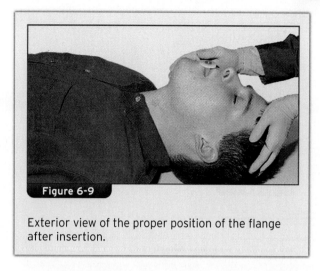

Figure 6-9

Exterior view of the proper position of the flange after insertion.

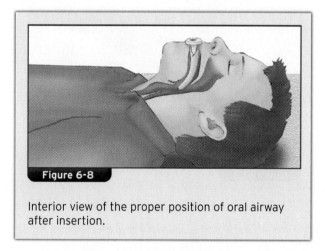

Figure 6-8

Interior view of the proper position of oral airway after insertion.

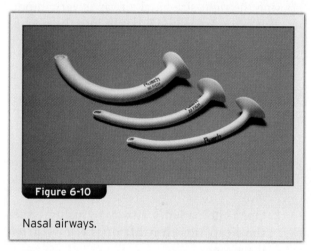

Figure 6-10

Nasal airways.

3. Insert the oral airway along the roof of the patient's mouth, with the curved tip toward the roof of the mouth **Figure 6-7**. As the tip approaches the back of the throat, rotate the airway 180° so that the tip points down toward the chest **Figure 6-8**. It should slip easily into the throat, with the flange resting against the patient's lips **Figure 6-9**.

If the patient is breathing adequately and does not have a spinal injury, roll the patient onto his or her side (recovery position) to avoid aspiration if vomiting occurs. Immediately remove the airway and have suction readily available if the patient regains consciousness or begins to gag.

Nasal Airways

A semiconscious or conscious patient who has a gag reflex can tolerate a <u>nasopharyngeal (nasal) airway</u> better than an oral airway. Unlike an oral airway, the nasal airway does not cause the patient to gag. It can be used on either responsive or unresponsive patients, but should not be used on patients with suspected fractures of the skull or nose.

Nasal airways are hollow devices made of soft rubber or latex **Figure 6-10**, are inserted through one of the nostrils and follow the nasal passage. Bleeding is a complication that can occur when a nasal airway is inserted. As with the oral airway,

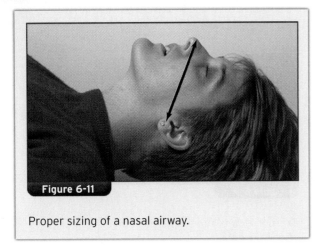

Figure 6-11

Proper sizing of a nasal airway.

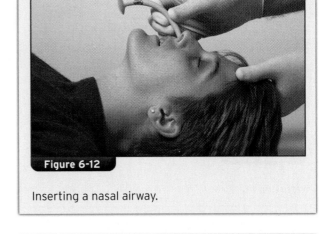

Figure 6-12

Inserting a nasal airway.

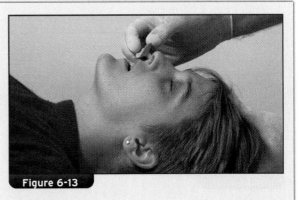

Figure 6-13

Exterior view of the proper position of the flange after insertion.

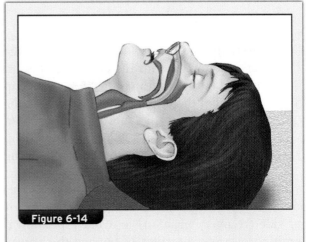

Figure 6-14

Interior view of the proper position of the nasal airway after insertion.

choosing the right size nasal airway is very important. If it is too large, it will not fit into the nostril. If it is too small, it will not keep the airway open or allow adequate air exchange.

Follow these steps when inserting a nasal airway:

1. Choose the right size device. It must fit in the patient's nostril. Measure the airway from the tip of the nose to the earlobe **Figure 6-11** . Alternatively, you can measure from the tip of the nose to the angle of the jaw.
2. Open the patient's airway by using either the head tilt–chin lift or the jaw-thrust maneuver.
3. Lubricate the airway with a sterile, water-based lubricant or with water or saline solution if no lubricant is available.
4. Insert the airway through the nostril, following the nasal passage straight back, not upward **Figures 6-12, 6-13, and 6-14** . Do not force the airway if you meet resistance. Instead, remove the airway and try inserting it into the other nostril.
5. Listen and feel for airflow through the airway.

▶ Ventilation Devices

Ventilation Masks

Mouth-to-mask ventilation can deliver an adequate volume of air to a patient if a rescuer ensures a tight

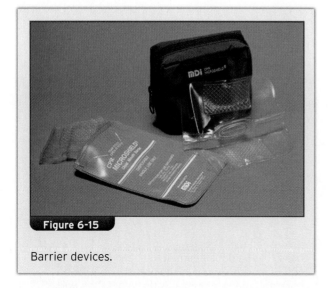

Figure 6-15

Barrier devices.

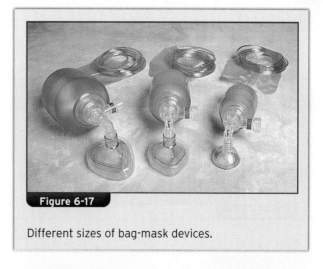

Figure 6-17

Different sizes of bag-mask devices.

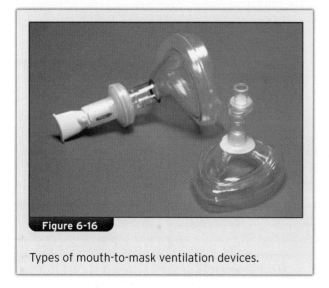

Figure 6-16

Types of mouth-to-mask ventilation devices.

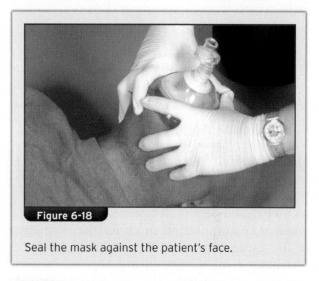

Figure 6-18

Seal the mask against the patient's face.

mask seal on the face. **Ventilation masks**, in general, offer some protection from infection. Certain types of masks have an inlet that allows oxygen tubing to be attached to the mask. No matter which mask you choose to use, you must consider a number of issues. The mask must fit well, have a one-way valve, be made of a transparent material, have an oxygen port, and be available in infant, pediatric, and adult sizes **Figures 6-15, 6-16, and 6-17**.

Masks vary in size and complexity from the simple face shield to the **bag-mask device**. Each type of mask has distinct advantages and disadvantages. Because you probably will not have the option of choosing the mask you prefer in an emergency, you should learn how to use all types correctly.

Follow these steps when performing mouth-to-mask rescue breathing:

1. Position yourself at the patient's head.
2. Open the patient's airway using either the head tilt–chin lift or the jaw-thrust maneuver.
3. Place the mask over the patient's mouth and nose.
4. Using both hands, grasp the mask and the patient's jaw. Press down on the mask with your thumbs, as you lift up on the jaw with your fingers. This will create a good seal on the mask and face **Figure 6-18**.

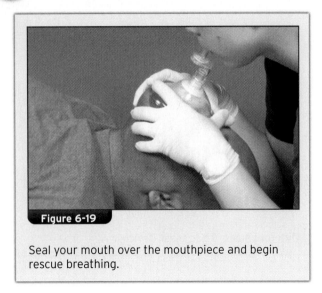

Figure 6-19

Seal your mouth over the mouthpiece and begin rescue breathing.

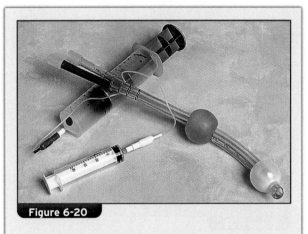

Figure 6-20

The esophageal tracheal Combitube (ETC). The ETC consists of a double-lumen tube and two balloon cuffs. The blue lumen is the primary ventilation port, and the clear lumen is the ventilation port if the tube is placed in the trachea.

5. Place your mouth over the mouthpiece and perform rescue breathing as described in Chapter 4 **Figure 6-19**.

Multi-Lumen Airways

Multi-lumen airways are devices that are inserted into the mouth without direct visualization of the vocal cords. They have been designed to maintain an airway and provide for proper lung ventilation when they are inserted in either the esophagus or the trachea. During CPR, you should remember to minimize the number of interruptions in chest compressions to perform the procedure. Commonly used multi-lumen airways are the esophageal tracheal Combitube (ETC) and the pharyngeotracheal lumen airway (PtL). The laryngeal mask airway (LMA), a single lumen device with a mask that protects the airway, is another effective rescue airway device.

The advantages associated with these devices include:
- Ease of placement (blind insertion).
- No mask seal needed.
- Protects the airway from aspiration.

The disadvantages associated with these devices include:
- Ineffectiveness if the cuff malfunctions.
- Requires proper assessment of lung sounds.

- Cannot be used on patients smaller than 5′ tall.
- Does not completely isolate the airway.

The ETC airway consists of a double-lumen tube and two balloon cuffs **Figure 6-20**. The blue lumen is the primary ventilation tube, used if the tube is inserted into the esophagus **Figure 6-21A**. The clear lumen is the secondary ventilation tube, used if the tube is inserted into the trachea **Figure 6-21B**. In the vast majority of cases, the ETC will enter the esophagus; however, if it enters the trachea, it functions as an endotracheal tube (ETT), with ventilations provided directly into the trachea and lungs. The clear cuff at the lower end of the tube seals off the trachea or the esophagus when it is inflated following tube insertion. The flesh-colored cuff near the middle of the tube seals off the oropharynx. Two pilot balloons correspond to the two cuffs. When syringes are attached to the pilot balloons, they inflate the two cuffs.

The PtL airway consists of two primary tubes (green and clear), two balloon cuffs, a stylet, a bite block, and a neck strap **Figure 6-22**. A third, clear tube passes through the larger diameter green tube. It contains the stylet and a cuff near the tip. The stylet is left in place as a plug if the tube is placed

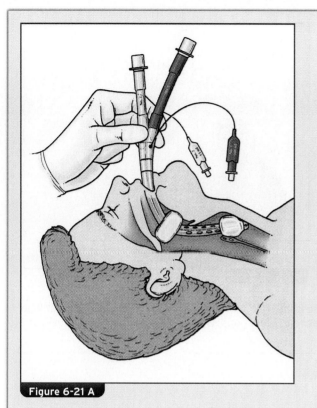

Figure 6-21 A

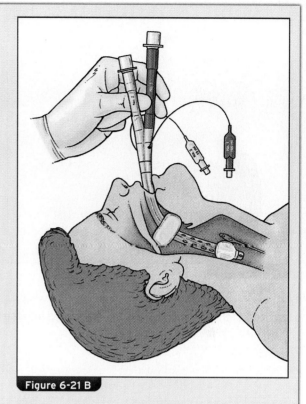

Figure 6-21 B

A. If the ETC is inserted into the esophagus, ventilations can still be provided to the patient. **B.** If the ETC is inserted into the trachea, it functions as an ETT with ventilations provided directly into the trachea.

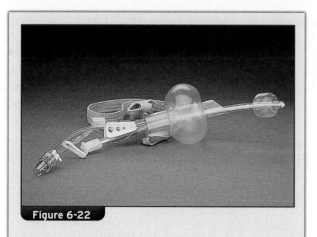

Figure 6-22

The pharyngeotracheal lumen airway (PtL).

in the esophagus, but removed if it is placed into the trachea **Figure 6-23**.

The LMA consists of a tube and a mask-like cuff at the end, that when in place blocks the larynx allowing air to enter the trachea only **Figure 6-24**. The LMA is inserted in the mouth and slid down the back of the throat until resistance is met. The cuff is inflated to seal the larynx, allowing air to go into the trachea.

Endotracheal Intubation

Health care providers must be aware of the risks, benefits, and indications of insertion of an endotracheal tube during resuscitative efforts. Insertion of an endotracheal tube may require interruption of chest compressions, which should be kept to a minimum. The health care provider who inserts the advanced airway should be skilled in advanced airway control.

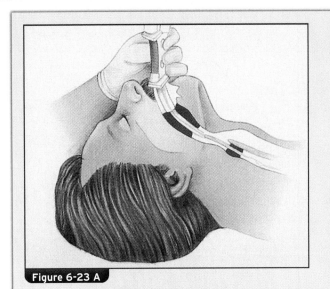

Figure 6-23 A

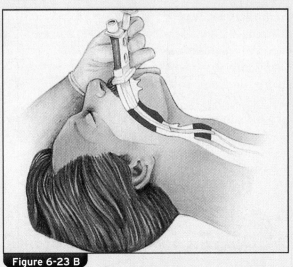

Figure 6-23 B

The PtL is inserted blindly into the oropharynx. **A.** If the PtL is inserted into the esophagus, ventilations can still be provided to the patient. **B.** If the PtL is inserted into the trachea, it functions as an ETT with ventilations provided directly into the trachea.

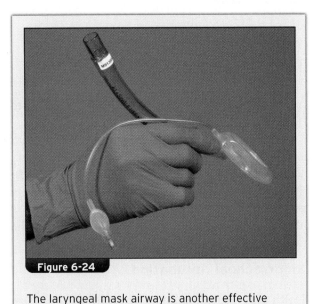

Figure 6-24

The laryngeal mask airway is another effective airway adjunct.

Once an endotracheal tube is in place, you can deliver continuous chest compressions at a rate of 100 per min, without pausing for ventilations.

Tube Confirmation Devices

Health care providers should perform a thorough assessment after an advanced airway has been inserted to verify correct placement. During CPR, you should minimize the interruptions of chest compressions. Assessment should include visualization of chest rise, presence of bilateral chest breath sounds, and the absence of sounds over the epigastrium (stomach). These techniques should be used continuously as needed. When transferring or moving the patient, it is necessary to confirm that the tube did not dislodge.

Exhaled CO_2 Detector

The exhaled CO_2 detector is easy to use, and its use is considered a class IIa action by the American Heart Association (2005 Guidelines). However, detection of exhaled CO_2 is not absolute as a means of confirmation during cardiac arrest due to low blood flow during a cardiac arrest. CO_2 detection during cardiac arrest is not a perfect means of confirming tube placement. More than one $ETCO_2$ device (eg, waveform, colorimetric, or digital) may be useful to confirm advanced airway placement during transports and when the patient is moved.

Esophageal Detector Device

The esophageal detector device (EDD) consists of a syringe that connects to an endotracheal tube. If the tube in not in the correct lumen (misplaced in the esophagus) the esophagus will collapse and the syringe will meet resistance and not be able to be completely pulled back.

Impedance Threshold Devices

The impedance threshold device (ITD) enhances the changes in intrathoracic pressures during chest compressions to increase both blood flow to the heart and blood pressures, improve circulation to the brain, and significantly increase the chances of survival after a cardiac arrest. The ITD, which is a small, lightweight device containing pressure-sensitive valves, selectively impedes the entry of air during chest wall decompression, providing an increased amplitude and duration of vacuum within the thorax. When used with active compression–decompression of CPR, the ITD prevents respiratory gases from entering the lungs during the decompression phase. By harnessing the energy of the chest wall recoil (ie, increasing the "bellows-like" action of the chest with each compression–decompression cycle), the ITD draws more venous blood back into the heart. This results in increased cardiac preload (the amount of blood returning to the heart) and, thus, increased cardiac output (the amount of blood ejected by the heart each minute), improved blood pressure, and enhanced vital organ perfusion.

Mechanical CPR Devices

Mechanical devices in theory will provide superior vital organ blood flow and increased blood pressures in comparison with standard CPR. They also benefit prehospital personnel with limited resources and can help prevent rescuer fatigue during CPR. These devices include the circumferential vest (an active compression decompression CPR device) and an inspiratory impedance valve (used in combination with the active compression decompression CPR device). The inspiratory impedance valve compresses the thorax using an automated mechanical piston compression mechanism and has been recommended to reduce the number of personnel required to perform CPR. However, no studies on the automated mechanical compression devices have showed an improvement in hemodynamic variables or survival in comparison with standard CPR. Health care providers and professional rescuers should evaluate compressions and ventilations just as they would with manual compressions. Even though these devices may improve hemodynamics or short-term survival when used by well-trained providers in select patients, there is currently no evidence to currently support the claim.

Bag-Mask Devices

The bag-mask device is a hand-held device with three main components: a bag, a valve, and a mask. The bag is self-inflating; when you squeeze it, it automatically re-inflates. The valve is a one-way valve that prevents the patient's exhaled air from entering the bag. The mask is similar to that used for mouth-to-mouth rescue breathing. The bag-mask device can be used with an oral or a nasal airway. The bag-mask device delivers a higher concentration of oxygen than a ventilation mask alone, approximately 90% to 100% oxygen when an oxygen source and reservoir are attached to it. Even without supplemental oxygen and an oxygen reservoir, the bag-mask device provides approximately 21% oxygen, which is also greater than the 16% oxygen provided by mouth-to-mouth or mouth-to-mask rescue breathing.

To use the bag-mask device effectively, you must practice regularly. The best results are achieved when two rescuers use the device. One rescuer maintains an open airway and mask-to-face seal, while the second rescuer squeezes the bag Figure 6-25 . The bag should be squeezed smoothly, not forcefully. Forceful compression of the bag, like forceful rescue

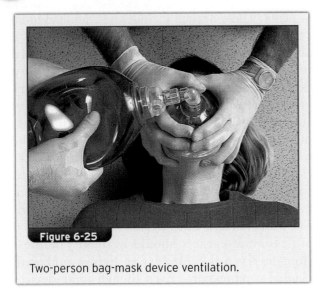

Figure 6-25

Two-person bag-mask device ventilation.

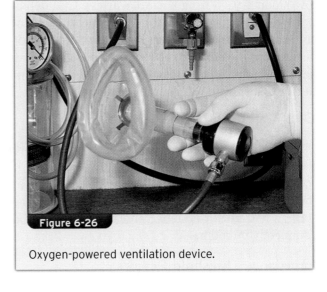

Figure 6-26

Oxygen-powered ventilation device.

breathing, will result in more air entering the patient's stomach than the lungs.

Oxygen-Powered Ventilators

Oxygen-powered ventilators are similar to bag-mask devices, but instead of squeezing a bag to force air into the patient's lungs, you press a button or trigger. These devices attach to an oxygen cylinder **Figure 6-26** . Like bag-mask devices, oxygen-powered ventilators can deliver between 90% and 100% oxygen. The advantages of oxygen-powered ventilators include delivery of a high oxygen concentration, protection from disease, and easy use. The major disadvantage is the need for an oxygen source to power the device. Once the oxygen is depleted, the device can no longer be used. Because the oxygen is delivered under a higher pressure, you must be careful not to overinflate the patient's lungs or cause gastric distention. These devices also cost more than the other ventilation devices discussed, and some the devices may not be appropriate for children. Consult your protocol guidelines regarding the use of oxygen-powered ventilators in your area of practice.

▶ Automated External Defibrillation

The most common initial cardiac rhythm seen in sudden cardiac arrest is ventricular fibrillation (V-fib)—an abnormal rhythm in which the cardiac electrical conduction system is in a state of chaos, resulting in an uncoordinated "quivering" of the heart muscle and the absence of a pulse. The most important factor for surviving cardiac arrest is early defibrillation. By applying defibrillator pads to the chest and administering a shock, you may be able to reestablish a normal cardiac rhythm. In the defibrillation process, a direct electrical current (DC) is passed through the heart to momentarily stop all electrical activity. The earlier this occurs, the better the chance that the heart's normal pacemaker cells will take command of the heart's electrical activity and produce a coordinated, regular heartbeat.

The time frame from cardiac arrest to defibrillation is a crucial factor in determining survival. The earlier defibrillation can be performed, the greater a patient's chances of survival. After 8 to 10 minutes of cardiac arrest, damage to the heart is often so extensive that the individual can no longer survive **Figure 6-27** .

Although not all cardiac arrest patients will need defibrillation, most adults who experience sudden cardiac arrest will be in ventricular fibrillation. For this reason, national efforts have been made to advocate placing low-cost, easy-to-use automated defibrillators where they will be most useful. These defibrillators, known as automated external defibrillators (AEDs), are now being

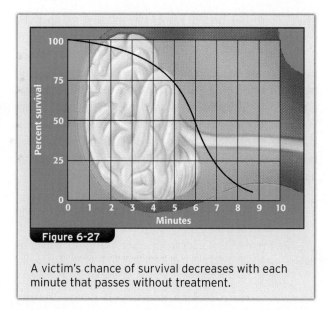

Figure 6-27

A victim's chance of survival decreases with each minute that passes without treatment.

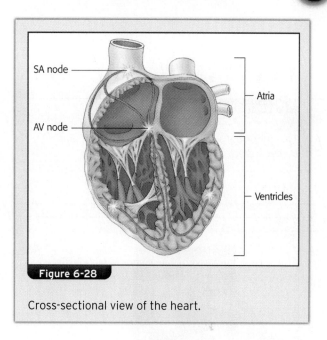

Figure 6-28

Cross-sectional view of the heart.

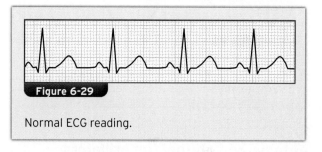

Figure 6-29

Normal ECG reading.

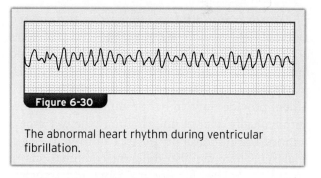

Figure 6-30

The abnormal heart rhythm during ventricular fibrillation.

placed in areas of mass gatherings—stadiums, shopping malls, factories, schools, and aircraft—so they can be accessed quickly when the need arises. Many law enforcement and fire department vehicles also carry AEDs.

The Heart's Electrical System

The normal pacemaker in the heart is the <u>sinoatrial node (SA node)</u>. Approximately every second it emits an electrical impulse that travels along pathways through the atria, causing them to contract. This signal is received at the <u>atrioventricular node (AV node)</u>, between the atria and the ventricles. The AV node acts as a relay station. Below it, the electrical pathway divides into two main branches, serving the two ventricles. When the electrical impulse reaches the <u>Purkinje fibers</u> in the ventricles, it causes the muscular walls of the ventricles to contract. This ventricular contraction forces blood to surge from the heart throughout the body, resulting in a characteristic pulse **Figure 6-28**.

Abnormal Electrical Activity

Ventricular fibrillation occurs when irregular electrical impulses originate from multiple sites in the ventricles. The heart muscle reacts erratically, trying to respond to too many signals. A chaotic ventricular rhythm results in the fibrillation, or quivering, of the ventricles, instead of a strong contraction. Fibrillation does not produce blood flow from the heart.

Another abnormal electrical rhythm is <u>ventricular tachycardia (V-tach)</u>. In V-tach, the heart beats at a rapid rate of between 150 and 200 beats per minute. At this rate, contractions become ineffective and the heart is unable to pump enough blood out **Figures 6-29, 6-30, and 6-31**.

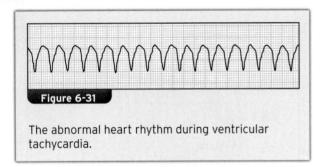

Figure 6-31

The abnormal heart rhythm during ventricular tachycardia.

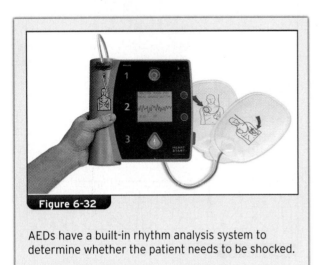

Figure 6-32

AEDs have a built-in rhythm analysis system to determine whether the patient needs to be shocked.

Automated External Defibrillators

There are many different models of automated external defibrillators **Figure 6-32**. The principles are the same for each, but displays, controls, and options vary. Some models have screens that display the heart rhythm and provide verbal prompts; others provide only verbal prompts. Some devices automatically analyze the rhythm, whereas others require the operator to press a button to begin analysis. There are also different combinations of recording devices for documenting and transferring patient information. Consult the manufacturer's recommendations for the specific model before using it.

The AED is only applied to patients who are unresponsive, not breathing, and without signs of circulation (eg, no pulse). Determine unresponsiveness, check for breathing, provide two slow rescue breaths if the patient is not breathing, and

check circulation. If the pulse is absent and the patient's cardiac arrest was witnessed by you, begin CPR and attach the AED as soon as possible. If the patient's cardiac arrest was not witnessed by you, perform five cycles (about 2 minutes) of CPR and then apply the AED. According to the American Heart Association, defibrillation success increases if 90 seconds to 3 minutes of CPR is performed before defibrillation in patients with unwitnessed cardiac arrest.

Follow these steps when using an AED:

1. Place the AED near the patient's head and turn it on.
2. Ensure the electrodes are plugged into the AED.
3. Expose the patient's chest and make certain the skin is clean and dry. If necessary, dry the skin with a towel.
4. Remove the adhesive backing from the two AED pads and apply them to the chest. Place the sternum pad on the upper right border of the sternum, so that the top edge of the pad is just below the clavicle (collar bone). Place the apex pad on the left lower ribs, below and to the left of the nipple.
5. Stop CPR (if in progress), do not touch the patient, and "analyze" the heart rhythm. Some devices require you to press the analyze button, while others do this automatically once the pads have been applied. The AED will now analyze the patient's heart rhythm. If the patient is in ventricular fibrillation or ventricular tachycardia, the AED will recommend defibrillation.
6. If defibrillation is recommended, stand back and make sure no one is in contact with the patient **Figure 6-33**.
7. Press the button marked "shock." After the defibrillation has been performed, immediately begin or resume CPR.
8. After five cycles (about 2 minutes) of CPR, check the pulse; if it is still absent, analyze the rhythm again.
9. Repeat steps 6 through 8 until additional help arrives at the scene.

If the cables or pads are not secure, the AED will give you an error warning. Likewise, the AED

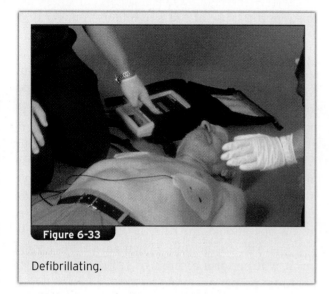

Figure 6-33

Defibrillating.

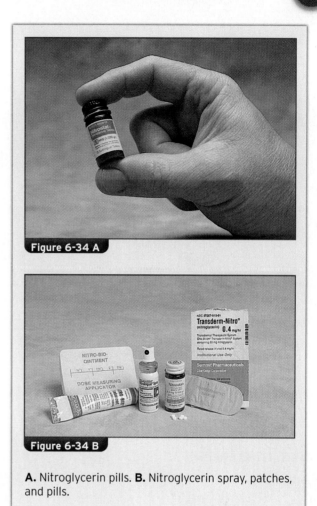

Figure 6-34 A

Figure 6-34 B

A. Nitroglycerin pills. **B.** Nitroglycerin spray, patches, and pills.

will not analyze the heart rhythm if the patient is moving, which is why you cannot use the device in a moving vehicle, such as the back of an ambulance.

If the AED states "no shock advised," but the patient still does not have a pulse, immediately resume CPR and prepare to transport the patient. This patient, as well as one who does not respond to defibrillation, needs advanced life support measures or has suffered too great an injury to the heart to survive.

AED Precautions

When using an AED:

- Do not use alcohol to wipe the patient's chest before applying the pads.
- Do not apply the pads over any medication patches, such as nitroglycerin **Figure 6-34** . Remove any medication patches with your gloved hand and wipe away any residue before applying the pads.
- Do not apply the pads over any implanted pacemaker or defibrillator. Place the pads at least 1" away from such devices.
- Do not attach the pads to any patient unless he or she is unresponsive, not breathing, and pulseless.
- Do not defibrillate a patient who is lying on a surface likely to conduct electricity (eg, in a puddle of water, on a wet sidewalk).

- Do not depress the shock button or analyze the rhythm until everyone is clear of the patient.

AED Use in Children

According to the American Heart Association, the AED can safely be used in children between 1 and 8 years of age. When using the AED on children between 1 and 8 years of age, you should use a dose-attenuating system (energy reducer) and pediatric-sized defibrillation pads **Figure 6-35** . However, if these are not available, you should use a standard AED. If both pads are too large to fit on the front of the child's chest, place one pad on the chest and the other pad on the back, in between the shoulder blades. Currently, there is no evidence

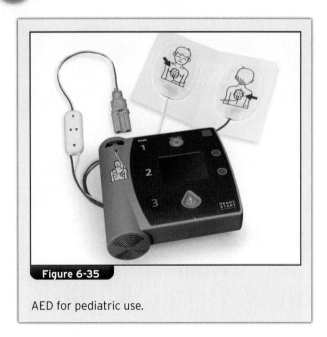

Figure 6-35

AED for pediatric use.

to support the use of AEDs in infants younger than 1 year. Follow your local guidelines.

Maintenance

AEDs can greatly improve the chance of survival for a victim of cardiac arrest if applied quickly and properly. But the device must also function properly when it is applied. To be certain that your AED will function properly when needed, you must inspect it regularly as part of preventive maintenance. Daily inspections should include checks to ensure all the supplies are on hand, the unit is operational, the batteries charged, and there is no damage to the unit. When an AED is turned on, it will perform a series of self-diagnostic tests to ensure proper operation.

Additionally, expiration dates should be checked on pads and batteries. Proper documentation should be kept of these inspections. If the unit should fail to function during an actual emergency, your documentation will be very important as the incident is reviewed.

► Ready for Review

- A patient's airway must be clear and open before you can begin rescue breathing. Airway obstructions may be caused by anatomic conditions, such as the tongue blocking the airway; this requires minimal effort to correct. Other times, the airway may be obstructed by foreign material such as food, blood, or vomitus.

- Manual and mechanical suction units are available to help remove debris from the airway. Mechanical suction devices are powered by batteries or pressurized oxygen, or are pneumatic (vacuum) devices. Whichever type of suction device you use, it is important to understand the machinery and not to suction too deeply or for too long a period of time.

- Patients can benefit from devices that help you maintain an open airway. If the patient is unconscious and has no gag reflex, you can use an oral or a nasal airway device. Select the correct size device to avoid triggering a gag reflex or blocking the airway. You can also use the nasal airway device on semiconscious patients and/or those who have an active gag reflex; however, do not use the nasal airway in patients with a suspected skull or nasal fracture.

- Various devices are available to support ventilation and reduce the risk of disease transmission. These devices can be simple ventilation masks, bag-mask devices, or oxygen-powered ventilators. The latter two devices can provide oxygen concentrations between 90% and 100% to the patient. Other devices designed to facilitate airway management and ventilation are multi-lumen airways, such as the ETC and the PtL.

- The single most important cardiac arrest survival factor is early defibrillation. The indications for using an automated external defibrillator (AED) are that the patient is unresponsive, not breathing, and pulseless. If the patient's cardiac arrest was witnessed by you, begin CPR and apply the AED as soon as possible. However, if the cardiac arrest was not witnessed by you, perform five cycles (about 2 minutes) of CPR before applying the AED.

- Once turned on and attached to the patient's bare chest, the AED will analyze the heart rhythm and advise whether or not a shock is indicated. If a shock is advised, ensure that nobody is touching the patient, deliver the shock, and immediately perform CPR for 2 minutes before reanalyzing the patient's rhythm. If no shock is advised but the patient is pulseless, perform CPR for 2 minutes and then reanalyze the patient's rhythm. Continue CPR and rhythm analysis until advanced life support personnel arrive.

► Vital Vocabulary

atrioventricular (AV) node A point midway between the atria and ventricles that sends electrical impulses to the ventricles.

automated external defibrillator (AED) A device that analyzes a patient's heart rhythm and recognizes the presence of ventricular fibrillation and pulseless ventricular tachycardia; advises the rescuer to deliver a shock.

bag-mask device Ventilation device with a face mask attached to a bag with a reservoir and oxygen connection; delivers more than 90% oxygen to the patient.

defibrillation Direct current (DC) electrical shock applied to stop fibrillation of the heart.

multi-lumen airways Advanced airway devices that are inserted into the mouth without direct visualization of the vocal cords; designed to maintain an airway and provide for ventilation when inserted in the trachea or esophagus;

prep kit

examples include the esophageal tracheal Combitube (ETC) and the pharyngeotracheal lumen airway (PtL).

<u>nasopharyngeal (nasal) airway</u> An artificial airway that is inserted into a conscious or semiconscious patient through one of the nostrils.

<u>oropharyngeal (oral) airway</u> An artificial airway that is inserted along the roof of an unconscious patient's mouth to keep the tongue from obstructing the airway.

<u>oxygen-powered ventilators</u> Devices that deliver, by the pressing of a button, between 90% and 100% oxygen to a patient.

<u>Purkinje fibers</u> Conduction pathways through the ventricles.

<u>sinoatrial (SA) node</u> Site containing the heart's primary pacemaker.

<u>ventilation masks</u> Masks of various sizes and complexities that are designed to offer some protection from potentially contagious body fluids.

<u>ventricular tachycardia (V-tach)</u> Rapid, regular heart rhythm that does not produce effective cardiac output; may deteriorate to ventricular fibrillation.

▶ Check Your Knowledge

1. An adult patient should not be suctioned for longer than:
   A. 5 seconds.
   B. 10 seconds.
   C. 15 seconds.
   D. 20 seconds.

2. When determining the appropriate size oral airway for a patient, you should measure from the:
   A. center of the mouth to the angle of the jaw.
   B. corner of the mouth to the back part of the ear.
   C. center of the mouth to the back part of the ear.
   D. corner of the mouth to the earlobe or angle of the jaw.

3. The safest and most effective method for providing rescue breathing to a patient is the:
   A. two-rescuer bag-mask technique.
   B. mouth-to-mouth technique.
   C. one-rescuer bag-mask technique.
   D. mouth-to-mask technique.

4. Which of the following ventilation methods delivers the highest concentration of oxygen to your patient?
   A. Mouth-to-mouth
   B. Mouth-to-mask with supplemental oxygen
   C. Bag-mask device with supplemental oxygen and reservoir
   D. Bag-mask device with supplemental oxygen and no reservoir

5. A nasal airway should not be used on a patient who:
   A. may have a skull or nasal fracture.
   B. is semiconscious with a gag reflex.
   C. gags when you insert an oral airway.
   D. is unconscious without a gag reflex.

6. When using an AED on a child younger than 8 years, you should:

    A. use pediatric-sized pads and an energy reducer.

    B. defibrillate three times in a row and then perform CPR.

    C. check for a pulse immediately after the AED defibrillates.

    D. avoid the use of a dose-attenuating system with the AED.

7. If you witness a patient's cardiac arrest, you should:

    A. perform 2 minutes of CPR and then attach the AED.

    B. call for help and perform 5 minutes of effective CPR.

    C. begin CPR and attach the AED as soon as it is available.

    D. avoid using the AED until the paramedics arrive at the scene.

8. You have attached the AED to a patient in cardiac arrest and have received a "shock advised" message. After ensuring that nobody is touching the patient and delivering the shock, you should next:

    A. assess for a pulse for at least 5 seconds.

    B. reanalyze the patient's cardiac rhythm.

    C. immediately begin or resume CPR.

    D. wait 3 minutes before defibrillating again.

9. The rescuer should not use an AED on a patient who:

    A. has a nitroglycerin patch on his or her chest.

    B. is not breathing but has a strong carotid pulse.

    C. has an implanted pacemaker or defibrillator.

    D. is younger than 8 years or weighs less than 55 pounds.

10. You encounter a patient who has been in cardiac arrest for an unknown period of time. What should you do?

    A. Perform five cycles (about 2 minutes) of CPR and then attach an AED.

    B. Immediately attach the AED and analyze the patient's cardiac rhythm.

    C. Perform CPR only and wait for paramedics to use a manual defibrillator.

    D. Avoid using the AED because the patient is probably not in a shockable rhythm.

Answers: 1. C; 2. D; 3. A; 4. C; 5. C; 6. A; 7. C; 8. C; 9. B; 10. A.

Special Resuscitation Situation

As a health care provider, you may find yourself in emergency situations that present special challenges. Although initial basic life support procedures still apply, special situations such as trauma, near drowning, hypothermia, and electric shock require additional skills.

▶ Trauma

Trauma is the leading cause of death for persons ages 5 to 44 **Figure 7-1** . To have the best chance of survival, a patient with serious trauma should be transported to the nearest trauma center for specialized treatment. But even with the best care possible, some trauma patients do not survive. This is especially true of trauma patients who experience cardiac arrest at the scene.

Whenever you encounter an unconscious person, you must consider the possibility that he or she has sustained a head or neck injury. This is particularly true of trauma victims injured by violent actions such as falls, motor vehicle collisions, or diving-related incidents.

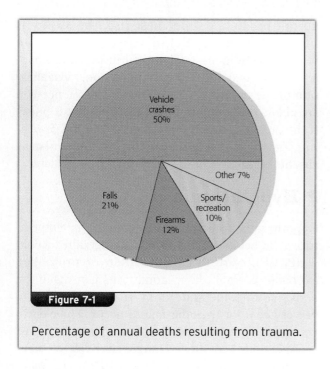

Figure 7-1

Percentage of annual deaths resulting from trauma.

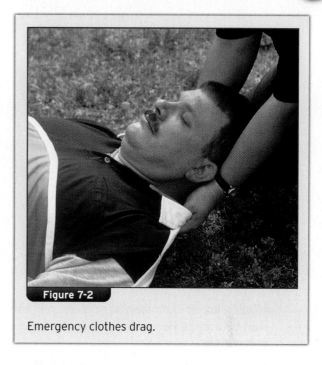

Figure 7-2

Emergency clothes drag.

One of the most common causes of unconsciousness is brain injury, but any serious head injury can also indicate injury to the patient's spine. Signs and symptoms of spinal injury include:

- Numbness, tingling, or weakness in the arms or legs.
- Loss of bowel or bladder control.
- Paralysis of the arms or legs.

Care

The care you provide to trauma patients begins with the ABCs. Start by carefully positioning the patient, keeping the head in line with the body if you need to roll him or her. Any unresponsive trauma patient's airway should be opened with the jaw-thrust maneuver; however, if the jaw-thrust does not adequately open the patient's airway, carefully perform a head tilt–chin lift maneuver. If you must move the victim quickly due to an unsafe environment, drag the patient head first to minimize the likelihood of additional injury **Figure 7-2**. Support the head on your forearms. Additional care includes immobilization with a cervical collar, head immobilizer, and backboard.

▶ Drowning

Drowning is defined as submersion in water resulting in death within 24 hours. Approximately 4,000 people die each year as a result of drowning. Near drowning refers to survival for more than 24 hours following submersion. For every person who drowns, it is estimated that four more are hospitalized for near drowning.

Water Rescue

If the victim is in the water when you arrive, you can attempt a rescue in one of four ways. Before attempting any water rescue, however, take precautions for your own safety. Never enter deep or moving water without the proper training, equipment, and personnel.

The four ways you can attempt a rescue are:

1. Reach the victim with an object such as a pole and hook. Make sure you have secure footing, and have someone grasp your belt or pants to keep you from being pulled in.
2. Throw the victim something that floats if he or she is out of reach. A throw bag, life jacket, or flotation cushion will do. Be sure to

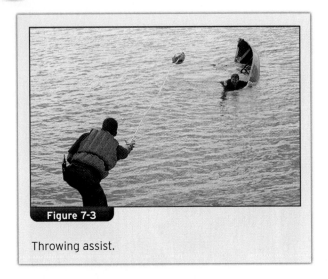

Figure 7-3

Throwing assist.

attach a line to the object so you can pull the victim in after he or she grasps the object **Figure 7-3**.

3. Row, or use a motorized boat, to reach a victim who is out of throwing range. Wear a personal flotation device whenever you enter a boat. Pull the victim into the boat whenever practical.

4. Go to the victim if the water is shallow and there is no danger to you. If the water is deep or swift-moving, you must have the necessary equipment and support personnel for a safe rescue.

Care

A submerged victim should be removed from the water as soon as possible to provide the most appropriate care. Although rescue breathing can be done in the water, CPR and defibrillation require the patient to be removed from the water.

Survival is uncommon in victims who have been submerged for prolonged periods of time; however, successful resuscitation with full recovery has occurred with prolonged submersion— particularly in cold water. Therefore, resuscitation should be attempted unless obvious signs of death are present (eg, decomposition, dismemberment).

Open the patient's airway and check for breathing. If the patient is not breathing, provide initial ventilations. If the chest does not visibly rise, reposition the head and try again. If both ventilations do not produce visible chest rise, the airway is likely obstructed. Begin airway obstruction removal techniques as discussed in previous chapters of this text (eg, chest compressions, visualization of the mouth, attempt to ventilate). Once you are able to ventilate the patient, check for a pulse. If the pulse is present but the patient is not breathing, perform rescue breathing. If the pulse is absent, begin CPR until a defibrillator is available.

▶ Hypothermia

<u>Hypothermia</u> occurs when the body's core temperature falls below 95°F (35°C). Immersion in cold water, exposure to cold weather, or prolonged exposure to cool, damp conditions can make the body's core temperature drop. It does not need to be very cold for hypothermia to occur. The elderly, young children, and alcoholics are particularly susceptible to this condition. In rare cases, people have survived extended periods of time without a pulse or breathing when their core temperature has fallen below 86°F (30°C). For this reason, it is important to attempt resuscitation even in extreme cases.

The signs and symptoms of severe hypothermia can sometimes be difficult to recognize, especially when weather conditions do not suggest it. Suspect severe hypothermia if you note these signs:

- Mental status that changes from disorientation, apathy, or aggressiveness to unresponsiveness.
- Lack of shivering. As the core body temperature drops and the victim becomes less responsive, shivering stops.
- Cool abdomen. The victim's abdomen beneath his or her clothing is cool or cold to the touch.
- Core body temperature below 90°F (32°C). This is not possible to measure unless you have an appropriate hypothermia thermometer.
- Stiff, rigid muscles, similar to rigor mortis.
- Blue skin; feels ice-cold.

Care

If you suspect hypothermia, move the patient to a warmer area, remove wet clothing, and cover the patient with layered blankets to prevent further heat

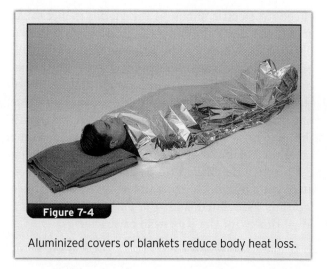

Figure 7-4

Aluminized covers or blankets reduce body heat loss.

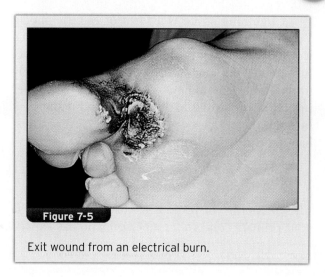

Figure 7-5

Exit wound from an electrical burn.

loss **Figure 7-4** . Be sure to cover the patient's head; this part of the body is a source of significant heat loss. When positioning the patient, do not raise the legs. This causes cold blood from the legs to flow to the body's core. Because severe hypothermia may dramatically slow the heart rate and breathing, the patient may appear to be dead. Therefore, assess breathing and pulse for 30 to 45 seconds before initiating CPR. Abnormal electrical activity (arrhythmias) may also develop in the heart. Handle the patient gently. Rough handling can cause cardiac arrest in a hypothermic patient with a slow pulse.

If the hypothermic victim is in cardiac arrest, begin CPR until a defibrillator is available—just as you would with any other patient. However, there are some slight modifications with regard to defibrillation. If the AED advises you to deliver a shock, deliver one shock and then immediately resume CPR. If the patient does not respond to one shock, focus your efforts on performing CPR, keeping the patient warm, and transporting to an appropriate medical facility for more aggressive rewarming.

▶ Electric Shock

Safety

Hundreds of people die from electric shock, including lightning strikes, each year. Although high voltage is clearly dangerous, deaths have been reported with household current of 110 volts or less. Safety is the most important consideration in dealing with

electric shock. When you arrive at a scene involving electrical hazards, take the following safety precautions:

- If you are outside, look for downed power lines before approaching the victim. Count the wires from pole to pole to make sure none are missing. Use a flashlight if it is dark. If the scene is not safe, stay clear and summon other professional resources, including the power company, for assistance.
- If you are inside, unplug or disconnect appliances and lights, or turn off the power at the circuit breaker or fuse box.
- If you feel a tingling in your legs and lower body, stop your approach. An electric current is passing up one leg and down the other. Lift one foot and hop back to safety.
- Do not move wires with a wooden pole. If the voltage is high enough, any object can conduct it.

During electric shock, electricity passes through the body along the path of least resistance, usually the nerves or blood vessels. The current may leave characteristic entrance and exit wounds, but internal damage may not be readily apparent **Figure 7-5** . A severe shock may also cause skeletal injuries, such as fractures. Any current may cause the heart to stop beating and go into ventricular fibrillation. If this is the case, proceed with resuscitation when there is no longer any danger of electrocution.

A lightning strike is a form of electric shock. Victims of a lightning strike may have burn wounds indicating the path of the current, or fractures from the force of the current. Victims likely to die from a lightning strike are those who suffer immediate cardiac arrest. Those who make it through the strike without suffering cardiac arrest have an excellent chance of recovery.

Care

The possibility of respiratory or cardiac arrest is your primary concern for a person who has experienced an electric shock. If the victim is in cardiac arrest, the heart rhythm is likely to be ventricular fibrillation, which can be reversed with early CPR and defibrillation. Because massive electrical injuries can cause fractures—including those of the spinal column—open the unresponsive patient's airway with the jaw-thrust maneuver. If the patient is in respiratory arrest, provide rescue breathing. If the patient is in cardiac arrest, begin CPR until a defibrillator is available. Unless associated with major bleeding, care for external burn wounds associated with the electric shock has a low priority for the patient in cardiac arrest.

▶ Ready for Review

- Special resuscitation situations include trauma, drowning, hypothermia, and electric shock. These situations present you with special challenges when providing care. Remember that trauma victims may have sustained spinal injuries, which require you to immobilize the entire spinal column.

- When water rescue is needed, you should attempt it in this order: reach, throw, row, and go. Never attempt a water rescue unless you have special training and equipment for this type of rescue. Consider the possibility of spinal injury in anyone found unresponsive in the water, especially shallow water. Clear the patient's airway before beginning resuscitation. Unless obvious signs of death are present, attempt resuscitation—even if the victim has been submerged for a prolonged period of time. This is especially true if the patient was rescued from cold water.

- Hypothermia may occur with patients who have been submerged in cool or cold water, and in other situations besides extreme cold weather. Because severe hypothermia dramatically slows the heart rate and breathing, assess the patient's breathing and pulse for 30 to 45 seconds before initiating CPR. Handle the hypothermic patient gently; they are at greater risk for cardiac arrest.

- When dealing with electric shock, make sure there is no longer any danger of electrocution. Your first consideration in an electric shock emergency is your own safety. Do not attempt to gain access to the patient until the scene is safe. Assume that patients may have serious internal injuries, even if entrance and exit wounds are small. Because electrocution injuries cause massive muscle spasms, you should also suspect a spinal injury.

▶ Vital Vocabulary

<u>drowning</u> Submersion in water resulting in death within 24 hours.

<u>hypothermia</u> An abnormally low body temperature.

<u>near drowning</u> Survival, at least for more than 24 hours, following submersion in water.

▶ Check Your Knowledge

1. To have the best chance for survival, a patient with serious trauma must:
   A. have blankets applied to him or her.
   B. be transported to a trauma center.
   C. receive oxygen as soon as possible.
   D. receive early care by paramedics.

2. Before attempting any water rescue, you should:
   A. take precautions to ensure your own safety.
   B. ask the patient if he or she can swim to shore.
   C. determine how long the patient has been in the water.
   D. have paramedics standing by so ALS care can be provided.

3. Severe hypothermia is characterized by all of the following, EXCEPT:
   A. a core body temperature of less than 86°F (30°C).
   B. severe disorientation or unresponsiveness.
   C. a lack of shivering as body temperature drops.
   D. relaxed, flaccid muscles due to a lack of oxygen.

4. The first thing you should do when caring for a hypothermic patient is:
   A. check for a pulse for 30 to 45 seconds.
   B. open the patient's airway with the jaw-thrust maneuver.
   C. carefully move the patient to a warmer area.
   D. complete a full head-to-toe assessment.

5. Which of the following statements regarding electrical injuries is FALSE?
   A. Electrical injuries may result in fractured bones.
   B. External wounds are a good indicator of internal injury.
   C. Ventricular fibrillation is common following electrocution.
   D. Deaths have been reported with a current of 110 volts or less.

Answers: 1. B; 2. A; 3. D; 4. C; 5. B.

appendix | Evaluation Forms

Student's Name: _____ Date: _____

One-Rescuer Adult and Child CPR Steps

No.	Task Steps	Satisfactory	Unsatisfactory
1.	Check responsiveness.		
2.	If unresponsive, activate the EMS system.		
3.	Open the airway (head tilt–chin lift or jaw-thrust).		
4.	Check for breathing. Look, listen, and feel for at least 5 seconds but no longer than 10 seconds.		
5.	If not breathing, give two breaths (1 second per breath).		
6.	If breaths produce visible chest rise, check circulation (carotid pulse, movement, coughing).		
7.	If circulation is present, but breathing is absent, perform rescue breathing (one breath every 5 to 6 seconds for an adult; one breath every 3 to 5 seconds for a child).		
8.	If no circulation, give 30 chest compressions (rate of 100 chest compressions per minute) and two breaths (1 second per breath).		
9.	After five cycles (about 2 minutes) of CPR, recheck circulation. If no circulation, continue CPR and recheck circulation every 2 minutes.		
10.	If alone and the patient is a child, call 9-1-1 (if not already done) after five cycles (about 2 minutes) of CPR. Then return to the child and continue CPR.		

Retest Approved By: _____ **Retest Evaluator:** _____

Student's Name: _____ Date: _____

Two-Rescuer Adult and Child CPR Steps

No.	Task Steps	Satisfactory	Unsatisfactory
1.	Check responsiveness.		
2.	If unresponsive, activate the EMS system.		
3.	Rescuer #1 opens the airway (head tilt–chin lift or jaw-thrust) and checks for breathing (take at least 5 seconds but no longer than 10 seconds).		
4.	If not breathing, rescuer #1 gives two breaths (1 second per breath), ensuring visible chest rise.		
5.	If both breaths produce visible chest rise, rescuer #1 checks circulation.		
6.	If no pulse, rescuer #2 performs chest compressions (30 compressions for an adult; 15 compressions for a child). Rescuer #1 gives two breaths (1 second per breath) during the brief pause in chest compressions.		
7.	After five cycles (about 2 minutes) of CPR, recheck circulation. If no circulation, continue CPR and recheck circulation every 2 minutes.		

Retest Approved By: **Retest Evaluator:**

Student's Name: _____ Date: _____

Responsive Adult or Child Airway Obstruction Steps

No.	Task Steps	Satisfactory	Unsatisfactory
1.	Determine if a patient is choking by asking, "Are you choking?"		
2.	If patient nods yes and cannot talk, give abdominal thrusts until the obstruction is relieved or the patient becomes unconscious.		
If the patient becomes unconscious:			
1.	Place the patient in a supine position on the ground.		
2.	Activate the EMS system. Have someone call 9-1-1 (or other local emergency number).		
3.	Open the airway and look in the mouth. Remove the foreign body only if you can see it. Do not perform a blind finger sweep.		
4.	Attempt to ventilate. If you are unable to ventilate, reposition the patient's head and reattempt ventilation.		
5.	If both breaths do not produce visible chest rise, begin chest compressions (30 compressions if you are alone or if the patient is an adult; 15 compressions if two rescuers are present and the patient is a child).		
6.	Continue visualization of the mouth, attempts to ventilate, and chest compressions until the obstruction is relieved.		
7.	If alone and the patient is a child, call 9-1-1 (if not already done) after five cycles (about 2 minutes) of CPR. Then return to the child and continue CPR.		

Retest Approved By: _____   Retest Evaluator: _____

Student's Name: _____ Date: _____

Unresponsive Adult or Child Airway Obstruction Steps

No.	Task Steps	Satisfactory	Unsatisfactory
1.	Check responsiveness. If unresponsive, activate the EMS system. Have someone call 9-1-1 (or other local emergency number).		
2.	Open the airway and check for breathing (look, listen, and feel).		
3.	If the patient is not breathing, attempt to ventilate. If the first breath does not produce visible chest rise, reposition the patient's head and reattempt to ventilate.		
4.	If both breaths do not produce visible chest rise, begin chest compressions (30 compressions if you are alone or if the patient is an adult; 15 compressions if two rescuers are present and the patient is a child).		
5.	Open the airway and look in the mouth. Remove the foreign body only if you can see it. Do not perform a blind finger sweep.		
6.	Continue attempts to ventilate, chest compressions, and visualization of the mouth until the obstruction is relieved.		
7.	If alone and the patient is a child, call 9-1-1 (if not already done) after five cycles (about 2 minutes) of CPR. Then return to the child and continue CPR.		

Retest Approved By: **Retest Evaluator:**

Student's Name: _____ Date: _____

One-Rescuer Infant CPR Steps

No.	Task Steps	Satisfactory	Unsatisfactory
1.	Establish unresponsiveness.		
2.	If unresponsive, shout for help or have someone call 9-1-1 (or other local emergency number).		
3.	Open the airway (head tilt–chin lift or jaw-thrust).		
4.	Check for breathing. Look, listen, and feel for at least 5 seconds but no more than 10 seconds.		
5.	If not breathing, give two breaths (1 second per breath).		
6.	If both breaths produce visible chest rise, check circulation (brachial pulse, movement, coughing).		
7.	If circulation is present, but breathing is absent, perform rescue breathing (one breath every 3 to 5 seconds).		
8.	If no circulation or pulse rate is less than 60 beats per minute with poor perfusion, give 30 chest compressions (rate of 100 chest compressions per minute) and two breaths.		
9.	After five cycles (about 2 minutes) of CPR, call 9-1-1 (if not already done).		
10.	Return to the infant and continue CPR. Recheck circulation every 2 minutes.		

Retest Approved By:	Retest Evaluator:

Student's Name: _____ Date: _____

Responsive Infant Airway Obstruction Steps

No.	Task Steps	Satisfactory	Unsatisfactory
1.	Determine if the infant is choking. Check for inability to breathe, cough, or cry.		
2.	Give up to five back slaps and five chest thrusts.		
3.	Repeat back slaps and chest thrusts until effective or patient becomes unconscious.		
If patient becomes unconscious:			
1.	Position the infant on a firm, flat surface.		
2.	Open the infant's airway and look for an object in the mouth. If the object is visible, remove it. Do not perform a blind finger sweep.		
3.	Attempt to ventilate. If unsuccessful, reposition the infant's head and reattempt to ventilate.		
4.	If both breaths do not produce visible chest rise, begin chest compressions. If you are alone, perform 30 compressions. If two rescuers are present, perform 15 compressions.		
5.	Continue visualization of the mouth, attempts to ventilate, and chest compressions until the obstruction is relieved. If not already done, activate the EMS system after five cycles (about 2 minutes) of CPR.		
Retest Approved By:		**Retest Evaluator:**	

Student's Name: _____ Date: _____

Unresponsive Infant Airway Obstruction Steps

No.	Task Steps	Satisfactory	Unsatisfactory
1.	Establish unresponsiveness.		
2.	If unresponsive, activate EMS. Have someone call 9-1-1 (or other local emergency number).		
3.	Open the airway (head tilt–chin lift or jaw-thrust).		
4.	Check for breathing. Look, listen, and feel for at least 5 seconds but no more than 10 seconds.		
5.	If not breathing, attempt to ventilate. If unsuccessful, reposition the infant's head and reattempt to ventilate.		
6.	If both breaths do not produce visible chest rise, begin chest compressions. If you are alone, perform 30 compressions. If two rescuers are present, perform 15 compressions.		
7.	Open the infant's airway and look for an object in the mouth. If the object is visible, remove it. Do not perform a blind finger sweep.		
8.	Continue attempts to ventilate, chest compressions, and visualization of the mouth until the obstruction is relieved. If not already done, activate the EMS system after five cycles (about 2 minutes) of CPR.		

Retest Approved By: **Retest Evaluator:**

Student's Name: _____ Date: _____

Automated External Defibrillator

No.	Skill	Satisfactory	Unsatisfactory
1.	Check for scene safety.		
2.	Check patient.		
3.	Check responsiveness.		
4.	If unresponsive, open the airway.		
5.	Check for breathing.		
6.	If not breathing, deliver two breaths.		
7.	Check for carotid pulse.		
8.	If pulse is absent and arrest was witnessed, begin CPR and attach AED as soon as possible.		
9.	If pulse is absent and arrest was not witnessed, perform 2 minutes of CPR and then attach the AED.		
10.	Call 9-1-1 if not already done.		
Defibrillation:			
1.	Power is turned on.		
2.	Electrodes attached to AED.		
3.	Ensure clean/dry skin surface.		
4.	Electrodes correctly applied to patient.		
5.	Clear patient.		
6.	Initiate analyze mode.		
If shock is indicated:			
7.	Clear victim.		
8.	Deliver one shock.		
9.	Immediately resume CPR.		
10.	After 2 minutes of CPR, check pulse.		
11.	If no pulse, initiate analyze mode.		
12.	If shock is indicated, repeat steps above.		
If no shock is indicated:			
13.	Check pulse.		
14.	If no pulse, perform CPR for 2 minutes.		
15.	Initiate analyze mode.		
Evaluator:			

index

image credits

Chapter 1
1-6 *Source:* American Heart Association.

Chapter 2
Opener © Photos.com.

Chapter 3
3-1 © Peter Willott, *The St. Augustine Record*/AP Photos.

Chapter 5
Opener © Brian McEntire/ShutterStock, Inc.

Chapter 6
6-29, 6-30, & 6-31 from *Arrhythmia Recognition: The Art of Interpretation,* courtesy of Tomas B. Garcia, MD; 6-32 & 6-35 © 2007 Koninklijke Philips Electronics N.V. All rights reserved. Reproduction in whole or in part is prohibited without prior written consent of the copyright owner.

Chapter 7
Opener © Index Stock Images, Inc./Alamy Images.